Praise for *The Millionaire Workout*

"If you're not healthy you can't enjoy life no matter how much money you earn. Exercise is an absolutely crucial piece of the health equation.

Exercise doesn't have to be boring and time consuming anymore because Ryan Lee has an amazing gift of creatively educating you on how to achieve phenomenal fitness. I have been exercising for nearly forty years and the first 35 years were almost exclusively cardio. About five years ago I shifted my approach to exercise and applied the principles he teaches and it has dramatically decreased my exercise time, while improving my strength and fitness level."

—Dr. Mercola
Founder of the World's #1 Natural Health Site: <u>Mercola.com</u>

"Ryan is the coach's coach. He is the first one I call when I have any questions. If you are looking for no-nonse business or fitness advice, listen very closely to what he has to say."

—Alwyn Cosgrove
Author of *The New Rules of Lifting*, *Men's Health* Magazine Fitness Advisor

---

"Wow! I didn't expect all the tips and tricks that work for health AND wealth! Ryan's terrific new book shows you how to achieve both in an easy to follow, step by step manner. Get this one!"

—Dr. Joe Vitale
author *"The Attractor Factor"* and *"The Key"*

"Ryan Lee has opened so many doors and given me so many opportunities it's been unbelievable. He taught me how to make an income online so I can free up my time and spend it doing things I would have never been able to do if I spent it in a gym all day training. The even better part is that's not all he did. When I do have crazy days with very little time to exercise his 4 minute workouts have been hard hitting and totally effective to keeping me energized and fit throughout the day. He has no idea how much he has changed my life."

—**Dan Grant**
Author of *True Weight Loss Revealed*

"Hands down one of the best success books I have ever read - and I've read a lot! If you want to reach your peak level of physical and financial success, you must devour this book."

—**Jermaine Griggs**
Successful Internet Entrepreneur, Founder and CEO of
<u>HearandPlay.com</u>

"Simply put - I went from a baseball coach to a six-figure online business. If you want to turn your dreams into realities, Ryan Lee is the man to show you the way."

—**Pat Rigsby**
Fitness Consulting Group, Inc.

"Ryan Lee is one of the few guys who practices what he preaches and lives a truly balanced life. I'm talking incredible income online, fantastic family and fabulous health! If you want to have it all - I'd follow exactly what he teaches you."

—Yanik Silver
Author, *Moonlighting on the Internet* and <u>Internetlifestyle.com</u>

Through Ryan's business guidance and teachings, in just a few short months I was able to launch a fitness bootcamp business which generates $8-10,000 a month, a coaching program where I taught trainers how to start their own bootcamp business, a teleseminar series where I interviewed 15 of the top health and fitness experts in the world and generated $35,000 in 7 days, and a "better body" coaching program teaching people how to achieve their best bodies in just 4 weeks, which brought in over $18,000. In addition, I have learned the quickest and scientifically proven methods to shed fat through his website SportSpecific.com and his Quatro Fitness DVDs and I use these metods to train myself and all of my clients. My entire fitness business and lifestyle are a testament to Ryan Lee and his expertise, and he truly cares about the success and well being of his students and followers."

—Scott Colby
Creator, __AmazingAbsFormula.com__ and __TheAbsExpert.com__

"Ryan Lee's passion for fitness and making money is utterly infectious. It is almost impossible NOT to do what he says and reap the rewards. I have traveled across country several times to hear him speak and own many of his products, I am never disappointed. Ryan has a gift for showing you what is possible, helping you believe that you can do it and then giving you very specific instructions on how to get there. If you are serious about getting fit and discovering how to earn more passive revenue, then read this book and do what Ryan says. You will be amazed at what you are able to accomplish in a mere 21 days."

—Valerie Waters
Hollywood Celebrity Trainer

THE Millionaire Workout

How to Get Rich Quickly and Stay Fit Forever... In Just 21 Days

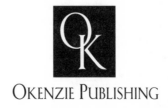

OKENZIE PUBLISHING

THE Millionaire Workout

Published in the United States by:
Okenzie Publishing
55 Kelley Green
New Canaan, CT 06840
Tel: 866-456-7926
www.okenzie.com

Book design and cover by Derek Brigham
Website: wwww.dbrigham.com

Cover photography: JC Taylor
Website: www.limnportrait.com

Manufactured in the United States
First Edition: November 2007

DISCLAIMER

This publication is designed to provide accurate and authoritative information in regard to the subject matter covered. It is sold with the understanding that the publisher is not engaged in rendering legal, accounting, or other professional services. If legal or other expert assistance is required, the services of a competent professional person should be sought. The authors and publisher of this material are also not responsible in any matter, whatsoever, for any injury that may occur through following the instructions in this material. The activities, physical and otherwise, described herein for informational purposes, may be too strenuous or dangerous for some people and the reader should consult a physician before engaging in them.

—Acknowledgements—

First I want to thank my wife Janet who has been right by my side for over 14 years. I am grateful to have found my soul mate. My daughters Jordyn and Lauryn who give me so much pleasure and make me constantly strive to be a better person. I am so blessed to have Janet and 'my girls' in my life. I cannot wait to welcome our 3rd child into this world!

To my mom and dad, who have always supported me and gave me the confidence to believe in myself. To my sister Robyn, Aunt Sharon, Cousin Danielle and all my family – thank you for being there. To all my friends (too numerous to name) thank you for you love and support.

To everyone who helped make this book a reality. Lou Schuler, who did a masterful job editing the book. I owe you, big time! Jayson Hunter for providing much of the nutritional information. Demetria Wallace who has been the backbone of this company - I couldn't have done it without you. Kerry Jacobson and the Collaborative Push team to helping make this book a reality. Zach Even-esh who helped a ton with the workouts. Sanjiv, Patricia and Mindie – I'm blessed to have you all on my team. Derek Brigham for a great job with the cover and layout. My friends and business partners Jim Labadie and Sammy See for their friendship and patience during the writing of this book. My A+ students: Alwyn Cosgrove, Brian Grasso and Craig Ballantyne – who took what I taught them and ran with it, and did it with class.

To all the people I've had the pleasure to know throughout the years. My first mentor Dr. Eric Small and all the staff and patients at Blythedale Children's Hospital. My students at Wildcat III. All my professors at Ithaca College. All my fellow track teammates and coaches from Clarkstown North to IC – you taught me the true value of teamwork. Chris Poirier and the Perform Better team for giving me a shot all those years ago. All the members of the PTU family – you guys rock. All of my online marketing buddies for their valuable advice with this book: Yanik Silver, Tim Kerber, David Frey, Jeff Walker, Russell Brunson, Joe Vitale, Roger C. Parker, Ryan Deiss, Joe Mercola, and Brian Sacks.

There are so many people to thank - I could spend hundreds of pages writing these acknowledgements. But there is one more person I want to thank.

Most of all I want to thank you - and all the clients I have been privileged to work with over the years. Without you, there wouldn't be a book.

Ryan Lee
The Millionaire Workout

—Contents—

Chapter 3: How to turn your knowledge, skills, or hobby into money. Lots and lots of money

Chapter 4: Six-pack abs for a seven-figure earner cash machine

Chapter 5: The Fastest Workout in the World

Chapter 6: The exercises Workout prep

Workout Prep

Total Body

Upper Body

Lower body

Core

Anaerobic

Chapter 7: Your 21 Day Millionaire Coaching Program

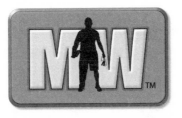

PREFACE

The Importance of Changing Diapers

I won't hide behind false modesty here: I've had a lot of success, I'm proud of that success, and I'm writing this book to help you achieve the same type of success. I run profitable businesses, I stay in great shape, and I devote more time and energy to my family than most guys in my position.

Currently, I run more than 50 websites. I've built three software companies, and published dozens of e-books, DVDs, and other information products. People have traveled all over the world and paid $3,000 to attend my workshops, where I teach them how to create their own products and launch their own online businesses. Many of my students have gone from financial distress to financial success in a matter of months. One, Patrick Beith, had eleven dollars in his checking account when he started using my methods. Within three months, he was earning more than thirty thousand dollars a month. (He makes a lot more than that now.)

As a trainer, I've worked with thousands of individuals of all ages and abilities since 1994, including college athletes at Yale and professional athletes through the United States Tennis Association. More than 120,000 people have used my online fitness products. That doesn't include the 24,000 fitness professionals who've attended my workshops, seminars, and boot camps, purchased my specialized products, or subscribed to my private newsletters. I was recently profiled in a cover story by *Millionaire Blueprints* magazine.

But here's something few people know about me: I don't possess any skills you don't have. In fact, I'm a pretty ordinary guy. I haven't set my alarm clock in years, and I'm the farthest thing from a workaholic. If I want to see a movie on a weekday afternoon, I see it. Most days I work from my home office, but sometimes I do my work from a chaise longue next to the pool. When I do go to my outside office, I get home in time for dinner with my family.

I've been married since 2000 to my college sweetheart, Janet, and we have two beautiful daughters, with a third child on the way. I've been changing diapers every day since Jordyn was born in 2003. By the time Lauryn, born in 2005, is out of diapers, I'll be busy wiping and powdering our third child. By the time he or she is potty-trained, I figure I'll have changed at least one diaper almost every day of my life for seven consecutive years.

Why am I sharing my diaper diaries with you? Because I want to show that we're more similar than different. We share the same goals and endure the same hassles. If you have the idea that you have to become someone else to achieve financial success, or that you have to compromise your commitments to your family or your health and fitness, I want you to get those thoughts out of your head.

You and I want a rich life, and for me, there's no point in being financially successful if it means sacrificing anything else that's important, starting with my daily involvement in every aspect of family life—right down to the baby's diapers.

While I'm on the subject of my family, I also want to make it clear that I didn't marry some Stepford wife who has no career or ambitions of her own.

Janet earned a Ph.D. in child psychology by the time she was just 25 years old. She's taking a few years away from full-time pursuit of her career to raise our kids, but she's still doing some part time counseling and testing with her own private practice.

In other words, we're a two-career couple raising our children together. We wouldn't have it any other way.

A Tale of Two Career Paths

As long as I've told you about my family life, I should tell you about my career. I wasn't born with any superpowers as a businessman, and no one handed me a magical formula for success. In fact, I began my career the usual way—at the bottom.

After I graduated college, I went to work as a recreational therapist and fitness trainer at Blythedale Children's Hospital in Valhalla, New York, where I worked with children of all ages and abilities for more than six years.

That job shifted my outlook on life in a profound way. I saw so many brave young kids facing death who still worked hard in therapy. They didn't want anyone to feel sorry for them. When you know that someone you've worked with and gotten to like is probably going to die by the end of the day, you realize how trivial most of life's annoyances really are. What's missing the latest *Seinfeld* episode or getting stuck in traffic compared to a good life ending at such a young age?

I didn't earn much—I lived in my parents' basement—but the hours were flexible and I had weekends and evenings free. That's when I started my first fitness-training company, which gave me an opportunity to work with healthy clients with a full spectrum of talents and ambitions—regular folks all the way up to elite athletes.

Naturally, as a personal trainer, I needed a Web site to promote my business. It was 1998, when most people had heard of the Internet but didn't really have firm ideas about what it was or how it could be used for profit. I confess it never occurred to me that I was staking my first claim in the medium that would eventually allow me to become a millionaire. I was just a guy with an active URL, trying to build a personal-training business.

But then a funny thing happened: As I began to add free articles to the site, I saw that people across the country—around the world, even—were finding out about it, enjoying the content, and telling people they knew about it. I was soon bought out by a large Internet company.

Okay, we all know how the Internet works, and we all know stories about small businessmen who became large businessmen when a big company came calling with an open checkbook.

I wasn't one of those businessmen.

I went to work for the company that bought me out. The job lasted all of two months before the company ran out of cash and let everyone go. Almost all of my compensation was in stock, so when the company went belly-up, the stock was worthless, and I was broke.

The timing couldn't have been worse. I was unemployed for the first time in my life, having left a safe, secure job at the hospital to experience the crazy world of Internet start-ups. And my wedding was just two weeks away.

I hit the pavement and within a week I found a job with another Internet company. I would start as soon as I got back from my honeymoon. This wasn't just a job to me. I'd be entering the corporate world for the first time. I was no longer a trainer with a website. I was a player in the most exciting and fastest-growing business opportunity of my lifetime.

But just 10 minutes into this new career, I knew I'd made a huge mistake.

The first nine minutes at the job were terrific. I couldn't wait to share my ideas on how to build our Web site with my new boss. When the meeting started, I rattled off one killer idea after another. She, with the skill of a seasoned tennis pro, returned every one of my shots with lethal precision. "No," she said, over and over and over again, until my ideas and enthusiasm were spent.

It was my first morning on the job, but already I could feel the clock ticking away on my corporate ambitions. Seven months later, I got called into the conference room, where my boss and someone from human resources were waiting for me. You know what happened next.

So here's the scorecard: After six years at one job, I was now unemployed for the second time in just nine months.

I was still running a few of my own Web sites, and they were bringing in some money. I tried my hand in the domain-name game with a site called domainrepo.com. That brought in about $1,000 a month, mostly through advertising and sponsorships. I also did online training through my first site, Complete Conditioning, and that brought in another $500 or so a month. Selling downloadable fitness programs generated an extra $200 a month. So I was doing okay, but wasn't making enough to live on.

This time it took me three months to find a job. The one I landed was at a new alternative high school in the Hunts Point section of the South Bronx. I was given complete freedom to start up a new health and physical education program for the school's poor and at-risk students.

It was (and still is) a very rough neighborhood. Here's an example: I parked my car right in front of the school, and yet my side-view mirrors and turn-signal lights were stolen three different times. Each time it happened, I went to one of the shops in the neighborhood to replace them. (I'm being generous when I call them "shops." They were really just run-down storage sheds.) When I told them what I needed, the proprietors would pull out a big black garbage bag filled with auto parts and sell me back my own lights and mirrors.

Needless to say, the job was challenging. Many of the young teenagers were actively involved in gangs. Some had arrest records. A disturbing number had already become parents. Still, I enjoyed my time there. I connected with a lot of my students, and I was happy when they came to me for advice.

At nights and during my free time, I began to work hard on my Web sites again. I launched my first paid membership site in late September 2001. (I was going to launch on September 11, but we all know what happened on that horrible day. Our school was right by the water, and we could see the World Trade Center towers burn and then crumble from our windows.) The Web site was an instant hit. Revenues increased for nine consecutive months. That's when I took one more leap of faith and left the world of paychecks and employer-provided dental plans to dedicate myself full-time to my fitness career.

It Wasn't Luck

You may have noticed that I skipped a few details. Like the many hours I devoted to learning and applying everything I could find about Internet marketing and promotion, or the thousands of pages of sales copy I studied to figure out what would and wouldn't work on the Web, or the fact I continued to work with clients as a trainer and coach throughout my years of full-time employment. What matters is that I learned a lot, and continue to learn, and the whole point of this book is to condense that knowledge into simple, actionable steps that you can follow.

Getting back to my story:

By mid-2002, my businesses were starting to pay off in a big way. I'd found a model that worked. Through my coaching, I was constantly coming up with new and better ways to help my clients, and I marketed that information in various ways on my Web sites. Before long, I was getting as many questions about how to make money as I was about how to get stronger or leaner. I developed products to help my fellow fitness professionals create and market their own products and services online, and by 2007, when I started writing this book, I had become better known for my entrepreneurial advice than for my fitness knowledge and coaching skill.

Still, there's one thing about my career that drives me a little crazy. I just hate it when people say to me, "Wow! You're really lucky!" It sounds arrogant to point out that luck had nothing to do with my success, so I rarely bother saying it. But I know the truth: I made a plan, I stuck with it, and I worked really hard.

I'd known since I was a little kid that I wanted to be married, have children, and be my own boss. I can even remember thinking how cool it would be to work from home, even though that was long before the Web existed and I had no idea what an adult could actually do that didn't require an office and a staff.

What I didn't know was how I could make any of my plans work. That's why I learned everything I could that I thought would help me. I didn't just study fitness. I also studied marketing, in hopes of figuring out how to create a business from my favorite pursuit. While my friends and coworkers were at home watching TV, I was at the library or a bookstore, reading everything I could find that might help me succeed. I even read books about success itself, in hopes of finding patterns in other people's success stories that would help me create my own.

I won't say I tried everything I learned. I won't say that everything I tried worked. Whether we're talking about fitness or money-making, some ideas that might've worked for other people won't work for you or me. I made mistakes and hit dead ends. But over time and with experience I figured out what works for most people most of the time. Now I want to show you the best of what I learned.

Meet Your Coach

When I sat down to put together the 21-day Millionaire Workout program, I didn't think about it as a book. Instead, I saw it as a coaching program.

When you think of a coach, you probably think of someone who trains athletes, or teams of athletes. Some of you, though, may visualize a career coach, someone who helps you make more money or advance in your profession. You've probably never encountered someone attempting to provide both types of coaching at the same time, for the simple reason that few fitness coaches have business experience, and few career coaches know their way around a gym.

But just because it hasn't been done doesn't mean it can't be done. After all, I've helped thousands of fitness professionals become financially independent, despite the fact that most of them had never taken a single business class. And I've helped thousands of unfit people become fit, including many who'd never found a workout program that worked for them.

So why couldn't I write a book that combined both topics into a single program?

I was told by several people in the publishing industry that I should focus on one topic. It didn't matter if I chose fitness or finance, muscles or money. The two topics are unrelated, they told me. Readers who're interested in one won't care about the other.

I don't believe it's that's simple. I've met plenty of people who don't see the point of financial freedom if it means you're so unhealthy you drop dead of a heart attack at 45. I've probably met at least as many who want to get in shape but are afraid it will divert too much of the time and energy they feel they need to devote to making a living. And everyone who has a family worries that devoting more time to health or wealth pulls them away from their loved ones.

More to the point, I know from my own experience that you don't have to make those compromises. You can be physically fit and financially prosperous and spend at least as much time with your family as people who aren't fit or prosperous.

That's why I decided to create a system that combines my two areas of proven success and expertise and shows you how to pursue both goals simultaneously.

Here's what I guarantee: Everything in the Millionaire Workout—every workout tip and every business strategy—has been used successfully in the real world. I've done all the workouts and used them with clients I trained and athletes I coached. They work. I've employed all the techniques I recommend for developing products, marketing them, and generating substantial and sustainable revenue from them. They work too.

Most important of all, they can change your life. In just 21 days, you'll not only start a fitness program, you'll see results and be well on your way to a lifetime of health-promoting exercise. In those same 21 days, you'll launch a business that can put you on the road to financial independence.

The 21-Day Program

Instead of filling this book with long-winded theories, I broke everything down into small, specific, easy to understand chunks. After all, even the biggest tree will fall eventually if you take a hard whack at it with an axe every day. Although small, each day's tasks are actionable, and move you closer to your goal. That's how you can create a business and launch an exercise program in just three weeks.

I've coached and observed enough people to know it's difficult to change ingrained habits in a day, or a week. That's why so many self-help programs, which seem so great the first few days, don't work over the long haul.

Each of the 21 days in *The Millionaire Workout*, which you'll find in Chapter 7, has its own section, with descriptions of the steps you'll take that day, explanations of why you're taking the steps, and finally a checklist to make sure you have everything covered by the end of the day.

The first two to four pages are your "Get Rich" plan for the day. This will tell you everything you need to do to launch a lucrative online business.

The next page is your "Get Fit" plan. It's your workout for the day. The fitness program will start off simple and easy, and then get progressively more challenging as the exercise habit becomes ingrained and your body becomes better conditioned.

The last page offers your nutritional goals for the day. I find that people are more likely to make permanent changes in their eating behaviors if they can tackle them incrementally, rather than all at once. All you have to do is follow one piece of advice a day and you'll be eating much better in 21 days.

Using the book is easy: Before you start the program, read Chapter 1. I'd also like you to read chapters two through five, but I know that a lot of you will want to jump right into the program. That's okay; I just want you to promise yourself that you'll read the other chapters as you work your way through the program.

What to Expect While You're Reinventing Yourself

When I sat down to create the *Millionaire Workout* coaching program, I assumed, for the sake of simplicity, that everyone would be starting off at the novice level in all three areas—business, fitness, nutrition. But I know that many of you are at different starting points. Just in the business area, you could be a complete novice who's never created a product or started a business of any type, or an experienced businessperson who's ready to try something that's more rewarding.

You may be looking to supplement your current income with a part-time endeavor, or ready to jump full-time into a lucrative online business that will provide lifelong income and financial security.

You may not have a clue about what type of product or service you can offer online, or you may have an idea for a business and just need a step-by-step system to get it rolling.

All of you will use the same 21-day program, but no two readers will use it exactly the same way. If you don't have an idea for a product, you'll come up with one, and by the end of the 21 days you'll know exactly what you need to do to produce it and start making money off it. If you have an idea, you can work on it over the next 21 days, and have everything in place to launch it successfully. And if you already have a product, by the end of the 21 days you'll have that product in the marketplace and generating revenue for you.

In fact, you can even do the 21-day program twice. The first time, you'll come up with the idea for a product or business and figure out how you're going to produce it and earn money. The second time, you'll launch your new business and start making money.

And, no matter where you are right now as a businessperson, you'll get into great shape—possibly the best shape of your life.

Ready? Let's get started.

1

EVERYTHING YOU NEED
FOR A SPECTACULAR LIFE

L et's begin by defining the word success. I came across a version
of this definition by Jack Canfield and it resonated so strongly
that I quickly adapted it for myself:

"To have the freedom to do what I want, when I want, as often as I want"

Success is freedom. Financial freedom. Being free from illness, sickness, or pain. Having unlimited free time. Which is nice to know, but it still begs the question: How do we get there?

Change Your Attitude and Your Behaviors Will Follow

Most self-help advice, in my view, is a Band Aid. It helps you stop the bleeding, but it doesn't heal the wound. It might even make things worse, in the same way a wound that's been poorly treated can get infected.

Here's what I mean: Let's say you're unemployed, broke, and sliding into debt. You get a job, so you're no longer unemployed. You've applied a Band Aid, and stopped the bleeding. But have you fixed the problem that left you unemployed in the first place?

Now, let's say you're sedentary and overweight. You start a diet and fitness program, lose some weight, and build some muscle. That's great. But have you truly confronted the thoughts and behaviors that led to the original problem? Do you now think of yourself as a fit, active, healthy person? Or is there a residual thought process that still belongs to your former self?

We've all heard of lottery winners who become multimillionaires overnight, but somehow manage to lose all the money and end up right back where they were. Similarly, we all know at least one person who's lost weight and gotten into a regular exercise program, only to revert to her previous habits, stop exercising, and regain all the weight.

The lottery winner might blame it on bad investments, greedy family members, or duplicitous advisors. My take is that he's pointing the finger of blame in the wrong direction. His financial thermostat was set on "low." When money dropped into his life, the thermostat temporary reset itself to "high," but that was so far outside his comfort level that he allowed himself to make a series of errors and miscalculations until it returned to where it was before.

Why would he do this? Well, put yourself in his place. Would you be comfortable with lots of money? Before you answer, ask yourself if you've ever described a wealthy person with phrases like "filthy rich," "greedy bastard," or "pretentious snob." The person in question may have deserved your scorn, but you also have to consider the possibility that you're uncomfortable with the idea of wealth, that you have a thought process that assumes large sums of money can't be made honestly or ethically. You aren't alone if you think that way. Movies and television routinely depict rich people in the worst possible way. From Gilligan's Island to Titanic, you see wealthy characters who're at best clueless, and at worst cruel, selfish, underhanded, and hateful.

The yoyo dieter might have similarly negative feelings about people who exercise, or about exercise itself. She may see people who work out as vain and self-centered. By extension, she may see exercise as a frivolous way to spend time. Even if she doesn't have negative feelings about people who work out, she might focus on the discomfort or monotony of exercise itself. The worst and most self-defeating type of thought process is when she sees herself as unworthy of being fit and attractive.

The people I've just described suffer from the same problem: negativity. I understand that there could be serious physical or mental health issues underlying a negative outlook; in those cases, of course I recommend medical help. But most people I talk to in my work suffer from you could call self-inflicted negativity. They've developed a toxic, corrosive attitude toward success without even realizing it.

The Five-Step Negativity Detox

A lot of forces work against you in our society. Unhappy people inflict you with their negative thoughts wherever you go. Unhealthy food surrounds you, and the more unhealthy it is, the bigger the marketing budget its manufacturer has allocated to promote it. Self-defeating behaviors are on display everywhere, while behaviors that promote health and well-being are dismissed as bland or excessively conformist, and sneered at.

If you were to approach this as an observer, rather than a participant, you'd be shocked at the sheer pervasiveness of negativity each of us encounters on an hourly basis.

You can't change the tone, but you can choose to ignore it. It wasn't easy, but I taught myself to do exactly that. You can, too, by following this five-step plan:

Step 1: End your media addiction

I don't have a 21-day program to accomplish this. I think the best approach is to cut off the media all at once. Cold turkey. Stop watching the news during the 21 days of the *Millionaire Workout* program. Stop reading the newspaper. Most of all, stop listening to political talk shows on AM radio and stop watching the shoutfests on TV.

I know what you are thinking. "If I stop watching the news or reading the paper, how will I know when something important happens?"

Trust me on this: If something important happens, you'll know. It'll be impossible to avoid. You'll see it in an email, or get a text message on your cell phone, or just overhear it in a conversation.

I haven't watched the news or read a newspaper regularly for more than a year, and I have yet to miss out on something important. I know if there's a hurricane coming (not an unimportant detail in my life, considering that I live in Florida). I know when there's an election.

I'm not saying you should forego your rights and duties as a citizen by not voting, or by remaining ignorant of the important issues in your part of the world. You can selectively find and absorb the information you really need without subjecting yourself to everything else.

You know what I mean by "everything else." How much information do you really need about the woman who just drowned her three helpless children? Like I said, you can't avoid knowing that it happened. You'll come across the basic facts even if you're trying to avoid them. What you don't need, and what you can avoid, are the minor details about her life that trickle out day after day, or the endless sermonizing about why it happened.

I'm sure you know people who get sucked into these big media sensations—the O.J. Simpson trial, the Laci Peterson murder, the never-ending saga of Paris Hilton. You and I both know people who ended up spending hours every day following these stories.

Honestly, can you think of any reason why anyone would make such a thing a priority in life?

Every now and then I revert to old habits. Not long ago, I listened to a radio talk show for a few minutes. The big news story of the day was that a major investment-banking firm had announced its annual bonuses. The average employee at the firm was set to receive something like $300,000, which of course is a nice chunk of change. I mean, who wouldn't want to get a check like that, on top of a regular salary that's pretty good to begin with?

When I heard the news, my first thought was, "Good for them!" I assumed they played by the rules, worked hard, and exceeded whatever expectations their employer and clients had for them. To me, it's like a pro athlete who has a great year and then scores a major raise in his next contract. It's about performance, and he performed.

But you'd never guess that the employees of that firm might've earned the money. The hosts of the show seemed outraged over the size of the bonuses, and the listeners who called in, if anything, were even more upset.

So I began to think about what the recipients of those bonuses would do with the money. Let's put you in that situation. It's bonus time, and you've just gotten a check for $300,000. And let's say that, after taxes, there was enough left over for you to fulfill a dream of yours and buy a bigger, nicer house for your family. Your bonus becomes the downpayment for that house.

Who benefits, besides you and your family? First, of course, is the family that's selling the house to you. Maybe they want to move up to a bigger house, or downsize to a smaller place, or need to move to another part of the country because of a job change. Your bonus has certainly helped them. The real-estate agents on both sides of the deal receive commissions, as does the mortgage broker. Attorneys and house inspectors get paid.

You also sell your current house, which means a dream fulfilled for the family that buys it. The Realtors and brokers and inspectors again get their share. So do three different sets of movers—one each for your family, the family you're buying from, and the family you're selling to. If you've ever bought or sold a home, you know that inevitably you and the buyers and sellers make repairs and upgrades and cosmetic changes. That means carpenters, painters, landscapers, roofers, and who knows how many specialists in flooring and windows and plumbing get paid for their work. So do the people who make and sell the materials. So do the people who make and sell you new furniture or appliances or whatever else you need in your new home.

Then there are the taxes you pay on all these transactions. You pay for schools, roads, libraries, recreation programs, police, firemen, administrators ... and that's just the local taxes. You've also paid state and federal taxes on the original $300,000 bonus.

Now, if you were the recipient of that $300,000 bonus, knew that you'd earned it for honest work you performed, and knew that so many people and institutions had profited from it, wouldn't it surprise you to know that complete strangers were complaining about it on a radio show? How bizarre is that?

Here's my challenge to you. For the next three weeks, do everything you can to avoid news in any form—TV, talk radio, newspapers. You won't believe how liberating it is.

Step 2: Beware the energy-sucking vampires

When I worked at the children's hospital, I had lunch every day with five guys from the maintenance department. They worked all over the hospital, fixing everything from the lights to the medical equipment.

They were fun to hang around with, but they were also overwhelmingly negative. They could find something bad to say about any person or situation. Moreover, they were proud of this peculiar talent, and happy to share their thoughts and observations with everyone they encountered.

After three months, I just couldn't take the negativity anymore. Even then, as a 22-year-old, I knew it wasn't good for my psyche. I could feel the energy and enthusiasm leaving my body like air from a punctured tire every time I was around them.

I didn't need to confront them, or create any drama. I figured it's better to be alone than surrounded by negative people, so I started going out for lunch by myself. I'd grab a quick bite, then head to the local Barnes & Noble to read for 20 minutes. It was a double-duty upgrade in my life: Not only had I gotten rid of a big source of negativity, I was using the time productively, to move my life and career forward.

Step 3: Drive and grow rich

If you've followed steps 1 and 2, you have some extra time on your hands. Now it's time to fill it in a positive, productive way. Let's start with one situation in which most of us are captive to negativity: our commute to and from work. The average person commutes 30 minutes each way. That's an hour a day, five hours a week, 20 hours a month, and more than 200 hours a year.

I highly recommend listening to audio books or motivational programs. You can learn more in an hour with a well-chosen audio book than you could in a month of listening to AM radio ranting. Plus, as a bonus, you'll never have to listen to a commercial.

Now, with one simple change, you've replaced the random negativity of broadcast media with positive, progressive steps toward improving your mind and your outlook.

If you look in my car, you'll find dozens of audio programs. I really like the motivational programs by Brian Tracy, Jack Canfield, and Anthony Robbins, among others. I genuinely enjoy listening to them. In fact, I might be the only guy in America who looks forward to the 20-hour drive from Connecticut to Florida with two small children in the car. I see it as 20 hours of information and insight I can absorb. (I should note that this strategy is flexible. More often than not, I'll listen to my programs on an iPod while my wife listens to the radio or reads to the kids. But if we feel like talking, we talk.)

I like these programs so much that I started producing my own. I have an ongoing coaching series, featuring interviews with business leaders, motivational gurus, and the most interesting and successful people I know. (For more information about the coaching program, visit **ryanlee.com/insider**.)

Step 4: Be SMART

If you want to reach your full potential, you must set goals. A great acronym for goal setting is *SMART:*

Specific: Be as detailed and specific as you can with your goals. Instead of saying, "I want to be fit," you can say, "I want to lose 12 pounds of body fat in 12 months by working out for at least 12 minutes a day, 5 days a week."

Measurable: You must be able to measure your results. For example, instead of saying, "I want to be rich," your goal can be stated as, "I want to be free of debt and have $500,000 in my bank account within 36 months."

Attainable: Is your goal within your reach? Wanting to become a millionaire might be an attainable goal for you, but is it attainable within the time frame you've allotted?

Relevant: Is your goal relevant towards your life purpose? Think long and hard about what you feel you're on earth to do. Does your goal bring you closer or farther away from your purpose?

Time-Based: Your goal should have a deadline. Never leave it open ended and pick a specific date you will reach your goal.

If your goals aren't SMART, they're really just daydreams. But if they are SMART, you can run every significant decision through a simple filter: "Is this action bringing me closer to my goals, is it a distraction from my goals, or is it just something that keeps me where I am right now?"

Step 5: Take complete control of your life, and keep control

After you've gotten rid of negative influences and gotten SMART about your goals, it's time to work on the final obstacle to your success: you. You must take responsibility for everything in your life. And I mean everything.

You have to give yourself credit for your successes and take the blame for your failures. You have to acknowledge that both are the products of your actions, or lack of action.

Are you in the best condition your genetics will allow? If not, why not? And when you stop to think about your genetics, ask yourself if you've truly maximized your potential. Are you fatter than your parents? If you are, then you have to assume the problem lies with what you've put in your mouth, not what your parents put into your DNA. You made the choices.

If you're unhappy with your job or the size of your bank accounts, you need to take responsibility for that. Don't blame the economy. Blame yourself.

Sometimes—and I'll admit this is a tricky area—it helps to take responsibility for things that may legitimately be out of your control. Bad genes happen to good people. I don't want you to beat yourself up over things that nobody in his right mind would blame on you. But I will say this: Blaming and buck-passing are corrosive. Taking responsibility is a liberating feeling. That's why, in my experience, it frees your mind and unleashes your creative spirit to take complete responsibility for everything in your life.

Five Bonus Tips

These tips aren't part of the program, but I've found them tremendously helpful on the path to success. (For even more tips, be sure to checkout my blog at ryanlee.com.)

- **Participate in a Mastermind group:** Find a group of four or five like-minded people, people who share your ambitions and attitudes toward success. Commit to meet on the phone at least once a month. You not only get to bounce your own ideas off your peers, you help them move toward their goals.

- **Act "as if":** Imagine you've already achieved your dreams. When you act "as if" you've followed through on your plans and reached your goals, you often get insight into how to achieve those goals. How would you carry yourself if you had already lost the weight you plan to lose? What would your posture be like? How would you dress? If your business plan had already succeeded and made you wealthy and influential in your field, what would you say to a writer during an interview for a local newspaper? If you were a speaker at a seminar, how would you address an audience of people who want to know how you got from where they are to where you are now?

- **Remember that money loves speed:** Don't procrastinate. I have one acquaintance who has been working on the same Internet project for almost four years. When you have an idea, take immediate action. Napoleon Hill once said, "Don't wait. The time will never be just right."

- **Double your output:** The best time-management tip I've even come across is this: Stop checking email so often. If you have an alert that lets you know when a new email has arrived, turn it off. Set specific times during the day when you'll check email. Here's the second-best time-saving tip: Put tasks together into chunks. Returning phone calls can be a chunk—instead of returning them piecemeal, return them all in the same block of time. "Chunk" your bills by paying all of them at the same time, rather than one at a time. Even if you pay some earlier than they need to be paid, you'll still come out ahead because you've used your time more efficiently.

- **Outsource:** Is there a part of your business that you don't like, or aren't particularly good at? Can you hire someone else to do it? It pays to outsource back-office tasks like billing or customer support, rather than taking them on yourself and running the risk that you'll procrastinate or do them poorly. Think of it this way: When's the last time you changed the oil on your own car? Or repaired your own computer? You could probably learn to do those things, but you probably decided long ago that it made more sense to pay someone else to do it, someone who could do it quickly and efficiently. Now extend that attitude to your business. You can hire virtual assistants or freelance IT specialists as easily as you can hire an accountant to do your taxes.

One Final Thought

My goal with the detox program and the bonus tips is to help you cut through all the noise and clutter of modern life, and by doing so take control of your life. Most of you should be able to act on these tips. But, as I mentioned earlier in the chapter, some of you will need professional help. (Remember, I'm married to a psychologist.)

If you have serious, deep-rooted issues, and feel as if you're always getting stuck in the same rut, please seek the advice of a qualified counselor or therapist. I truly want to help you get the most out of life. If you aren't able to act on all the steps of my coaching program, it won't work. [MW]

II

How to Create a 24-Hour-a-Day, Seven-Day-a-Week Cash Machine

I'm not a financial guru, I don't have an Ivy League MBA, and I've never worked as a financial planner. What I have is real-world experience. I've built a handful of successful businesses on the Internet with start-up costs of less than $100 per venture. If I wanted to, I could stop working today and live comfortably off the income from those businesses for the rest of my life.

I'm not knocking higher education. I have a master's degree in exercise physiology, which has helped me become a better trainer and coach. I'm married to a woman with a Ph.D. in her field, as I've mentioned. But if you have any notion that you need specialized education or training in business or finance to succeed as an entrepreneur, I want to convince you otherwise.

Here's a story from my own graduate studies that helps illustrate my point:

I went to night school for three years to earn my master's degree. As my time in the program was coming to a close, I had an interesting conversation with my exercise physiology professor.

By that time, I was already generating income selling coaching programs and information products on the Internet. My professor, as it happens, had recently produced his own DVD, but he'd lost money on the deal. And here he was asking me for advice after class.

My professor, of course, was an expert in exercise science, not finance. Still, I was surprised that he hadn't done any research into marketing before he produced and tried to sell his product.

That's when I realized that if I wanted to make more money, I'd have to seek out the people who've done what I wanted to do. I'd have to buy their programs, attend their seminars, perhaps even hire them to coach me. In other words, I needed to stop modeling unsuccessful people, and study the ones who've done what I wanted to do.

Boy, did it work.

I've gone from a recreational therapist making $26,000 a year and living in my parents' basement to a millionaire. I did it by studying other successful people and taking *immediate* action on my ideas.

My Big Discovery: It's Not What You Make, It's What You Keep

At the time of that discussion with my professor, I approached income and employment the way most people do. I concentrated on my full-time job and I made extra money by trading hours for dollars as a personal trainer. I made money when I worked. I didn't make money when I wasn't working—when I was eating, sleeping, studying for my master's degree, or spending time with my wife. Like almost everyone else, my potential to make money was limited by the number of hours I could work and the amount of money I could persuade other people to pay me.

In one of my grad-school classes, the assignment was to plan out a business we'd like to run. At the time, I wanted to open a personal-training studio. So I did the required research, visited a few facilities, and ran the numbers.

Those numbers told me the business didn't make much sense.

Start-up costs would be $50,000 to $100,000, and that was for a small studio. A bigger, more ambitious set-up could cost millions—all before I'd signed up a single member or trained a single client.

It would take years for a commercial gym or personal-training studio to turn a profit, and there was no guarantee it would ever happen. Even in successful gyms, the margins were razor-thin; a few clients flaking out, an unexpected lawsuit, or some other random instance of bad luck could mean the difference between black ink and red. And that was if you did everything right. Make a few mistakes, as all entry-level businesspeople will do, and you could lose every penny of your investment, leaving you with a stack of unpaid bills that might take years to pay off.

At the time I was taking the class and doing this research, I'd already launched my first Internet business for less than $50. I wasn't getting rich, but I'd been operating in the black from the first week.

You don't need an MBA or a Ph.D. in statistics to see how important it is to keep overhead as low as possible. I ran the business by myself from my home, so I didn't have to pay anybody or take on the burden of a lease. In fact, I didn't have any employees for my first four years in business.

So I dropped the fantasy of having my own training facility. I learned more about information marketing, and realized that it really is the perfect business. Here's why:

- **I can work from anywhere.** I started my first Internet business from my parents' basement. Now, with a wireless modem, I can write information products by the pool, or answer emails from a bookstore. I can travel almost anywhere in the world and run my businesses from any place with Internet access. Wherever I am, there's my office.

- **I can launch new businesses with almost no costs.** All I need is an idea, a URL, and a mailing list. If I produce a good product or offer a good service, I make money. If the idea or my execution of it misfires, I can learn from my mistake and move on to the next idea without sacrificing any of the money I've earned from the ideas that worked.

- **My customers can buy my products and services no matter where they live,** as I realized back in 1999, when I got an email from the United Kingdom. Someone in London was asking me questions about training. I found that mind boggling. If I'd opened that training studio, I'd be limited to clients who lived within driving distance. Today, I have customers in 32 different countries.

- **Once I have a product or service that works—that was well-conceived, well-executed, and well-marketed—I can make money from that product 24 hours a day, seven days a week.** There is no limit to the amount of money I can generate from a single product. And there's no limit to the number of businesses I can run simultaneously.

You Too Can Play This Game

As I said in the preface to The Millionaire Workout, I don't have any special genius that allows me to run my businesses with low overhead and big returns. You can produce a downloadable book that costs you virtually nothing beyond your time and effort. You can charge whatever you think your target audience is willing to pay—$5, $100, or anything in between. That's with no office expenses, no employees, no inventory, and no fulfillment costs. Almost every penny you make is profit.

Turn the page, and I'll show you how.

III

How to Turn Your Knowledge, Skills, or Hobbies Into Money – Lots and Lots of Money

At this point, I wouldn't blame you if you entertained the thought that I might not be completely sane. We've all been conditioned to look at our knowledge, skills, and interests as commodities we can rent out to a finite number of clients in a circumscribed geographic area. We see our best assets as having limited worth, because they're of limited value to our employer or clients. They're worth whatever this small circle of people says they're worth.

But I can promise you this: You know something that other people don't. Everyone has some type of specialized information, or has a talent for finding specialized information, that other people want and are willing to purchase. I've spoken with thousands of people who wanted to know more about creating information products, and I've yet to meet anyone who had nothing to offer. There's *always* something you can turn into an information product.

A few weeks before I wrote this chapter, my wife and I attended a wedding in upstate Connecticut. A guy at our table told us he installs car stereos for a living. He works two jobs to support his family, which includes a newborn son. My first thought was, this guy could make some terrific information products. I could see him creating a series of DVDs teaching people how to do it themselves. Or publishing a private newsletter for industry technicians, where they could share news about what they do, and strategies for doing it better or more profitably. My second thought was, he could make enough money off these products that he wouldn't need to work that second job. Maybe he could do so well that he wouldn't need the first job. I've seen it happen more times than I could ever count.

Here are some more examples of how you can profit from the information you already have. I'm going to use extremely specific examples, but each one applies to a broad range of similar jobs. The suggestions I offer for an electronics salesman who specializes in home-theater equipment could apply to any type of salesman with a specialty. Similarly, anybody who builds or repairs things—from electricians to pastry chefs—should be able to use variations on the suggestions I make for a handyman in the second example.

Electronics salesperson

Let's say you work the floor at a big electronics retailer. The store sells everything from cell phones to high-definition televisions, but you've developed a specialty in home theaters. You're good at selling them. And because you've been dealing with the public for a long time, you've started to see some patterns in the types of questions they ask and the concerns they express. So your first option for an information product could be something that helps these consumers.

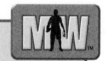

Topic 1: "How to set up and get the most out of your new home theater"

Market: people who buy sophisticated audio and video equipment but don't understand how it works and quickly become frustrated with the products and their own inability to use them in a way that justifies the money they've spent

What they want: to learn how to set up the home theater; to get the most out of it once it's set up properly; and to be able to trouble-shoot the problems that inevitably arise

Potential information products: manuals, DVDs, e-books

Yes, the products themselves come with installation manuals. And there's no shortage of magazines and books for electronics aficionados who're always looking for the latest, greatest stuff. But think about your own experience with owner's manuals. Are they simple, clear, and easy to use? Maybe you understand what they're trying to say, but chances are your customers find them infuriating. Now think about the products that appeal to audio and video buffs. Aren't they way over the head of the average consumer, the person who's mystified by the instruction booklet?

So you see a potential gap in the information marketplace. The person who isn't handy, who doesn't have an intuitive feel for electronics, gets little from the existing material. The product that speaks directly to that person and addresses his most pressing concerns probably doesn't yet exist, and won't exist until you create it.

But maybe you're more interested in helping your fellow salespeople than you are in addressing the concerns of your customers. In that case ...

Topic 2: "How to improve your sales of big-ticket electronics by 50 percent"

Market: store managers, commission-based salespeople

What they want: to improve sales

Potential information products: audio CDs (which they can listen to on the way to work), workbooks, seminars

---

Again, there's lots of material about how to understand consumers and how to be a better salesman. You should already be familiar with it. But is there a book or product that specifically addresses people like you, who make a living selling a specific type of product? If not, you could be the one to create it.

I put seminars on the list of potential products. If you're a good salesman, you're probably a good public speaker. And people in your profession probably respond to person-to-person instruction better than textbooks. So this is a great opportunity to hit the road and speak to groups of salespeople. In most cases, their employers will pay for them to attend your seminars, since the employers have the most to gain.

One last audience to consider: people who want to purchase the type of products you sell but are fearful of the process.

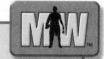

Topic 3: "How to buy the perfect home theater without getting ripped off"

Market: people who have the money and desire to buy high-end electronics, but worry that their lack of knowledge about the products will make them easy marks for unscrupulous retailers

What they want: confidence that they will get the best products for their needs, at the best price

Potential information products: pamphlet, book, e-book

This person probably wants something short, simple, straightforward, and up to date. (The beauty of products like e-books, which I'll discuss in more detail at the end of this chapter, is that they can be updated constantly without leaving you with a garage full of obsolete books or pamphlets.)

Since this customer fears people like you, you'll give her courage in the form of a product that reveals all the dirty tricks of your profession. And yes, your profession has dirty tricks; every trade does. I'm a trainer, and I could tell you stories about people in my field that would give you nightmares.

She needs simple guidelines that help her narrow her choices, so tell her how much power she needs for the space she has, what types of optional equipment improve the picture or sound, what stuff is useless but will get pushed at her anyway, and how much money she should expect to spend.

There's also information that would be helpful but that she wouldn't think to seek out. So tell her the best time of year to buy these products, what brands have better track records than others, and what "code words" she can use to tip off a salesperson that she isn't an easy mark for unscrupulous tactics.

You may need to do this type of product anonymously, so you don't jeopardize your current job. In fact, anonymity could give the product more value, since it tells your customer that she's getting information so valuable, and so closely guarded, that you'd get fired if your boss found out you were spilling the secrets only insiders are supposed to know.

Handyman

As someone with a broad background in repairing all the things that break, you have an easy and natural transition into information products. Fewer homeowners these days know how to fix anything; our natural inclination is to panic the minute something starts to creak, leak, or crack. So you have two big market opportunities: people who want to learn how to do it themselves, and people who are good with their hands and want to get into the business you're already in.

Topic 1: "How to quickly and easily fix your own ..."

Market: homeowners who can't afford to hire someone every time something snaps; homeowners who can afford it but don't want to pay someone out of principle; entry-level landlords who own a small number of rental properties and whose profit margins disappear every time they have to call a professional to fix something a tenant has broken; people who live out in the middle of nowhere and have a hard time getting anyone to come out for minor household work

What they want: to save money on basic household repairs, and to feel empowered with the knowledge that they can fix things

Potential information products: how-to manuals; DVDs; seminars

Home Depot and Lowe's have shelves full of books on home repair, and offer seminars for homeowners. So what can you do that they can't? You can explain how to do the work faster, or with less expense. You can show insider's secrets and shortcuts. You can appeal to new-home buyers by showing simple and inexpensive ways to make their home more functional, or go the other direction and show people trying to sell a home how to make it appear more cozy or luxurious.

The key here is to use your personal experiences as a handyman to understand what people want that they can't get from the materials that already exist. Are they looking for projects that improve home value? Increase storage space? Allow them to heat or cool their homes with less energy? Just about any concern a client expresses to you could be the basis for an information product.

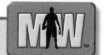

Topic 2: "How to make money as a handyman"

Market: people who enjoy fixing and improving things and want to know how to make a living at it; people who already have a full-time job and are looking for a way to earn part-time income

What they want: straightforward, actionable information on how to go from being good with their hands to making money doing what they enjoy

Potential information products: how-to manuals; DVDs; seminars and workshops

Whatever information product you start off with should work to your strengths. If you're good at articulating your ideas and explaining how to make them work, then you'll probably be able to produce useful how-to manuals and be comfortable speaking at your seminars. Are you a natural teacher? Consider offering workshops. If you're more comfortable doing than explaining, DVDs would probably work best for you.

How to Make Money from Your Hobbies

By now, you might be thinking that the two examples I offered don't have anything to do with you. You aren't a talented, experienced salesperson with a lucrative specialty. You aren't someone who has the skills of a handyman. Maybe you've bounced around from job to job and don't think you have any specialized knowledge or talent that you can teach others.

Get that thought out of your head. There's always something you know or can do better than other people. *Always.*

If your profession offers no obvious possibilities, look at your hobbies. What do you like to do? Put another way: When you're at work, what do you wish you could be doing instead? What do you most look forward to doing outside of work? What do you love to talk about when you're out with friends and family? What topic can you go on and on about for hours? In what area of knowledge do people who know you come to you for advice?

Maybe you love to shop. If so, you've probably learned a lot about shopping without realizing it. You can teach others where to find the most valuable coupons, when retailers have their best sales of the year for a variety of categories (clothes, cars, electronics), or how to find second-hand shops that offer the highest-quality, least-used stuff that other people bought but didn't bother taking out of the box. Because you love to shop, you've figured out how to get bargains that are invisible to almost everyone else. That means you can create an information product that shows other shoppers what only the truly obsessed shoppers would know or could easily find out.

Let's say you're a fashion buff. You spend your free time flipping through fashion magazines, and challenge yourself to recreate those looks for a fraction of the price. Sometimes you find ways to improve on what you see in the magazines. Your friends come to you for advice on what to wear and how to wear it. It doesn't matter if you're an intern or a CEO—if you have this kind of fashion sense, and you gained it despite the fact no one paid you to have it, you can create information products. You can teach people how to dress better than they do now—which fabrics and patterns look good together, and which should never be seen on the same body at the same time. You can help people with different body types find clothes that fit better and are more flattering. No, you aren't a big-name designer or a buyer for a major department-store chain or a writer for Vogue or GQ. But you probably have a better grasp on the sartorial dilemmas of people like you than the highly paid, highly visible fashion elite.

Or you could mix and match within these two categories, and exploit specialties within specialties. Maybe you're an obsessed shopper who's particularly obsessed with fashion. Or you're a fashion hound who's particularly good with children's outfits. If you love it, you're good at it, and your friends ask for your advice about it, you can create an information product on that topic.

Some more general topic areas where you might have some expertise:

- Academics (standardized-test prep; how to get into a specific college or type of college; best preschools for a variety of incomes and preferences; guides to tutors who live in your area)

- Athletics (sports skills; coaching; sport-specific conditioning; best schools and camps to improve sports skills)

- Collectibles (how to become a collector with a particular specialty, such as baseball cards, stamps, coins, or antiques; how to sell a collection you inherited; how to buy or sell collectibles on eBay without getting ripped off)

- Computer skills (Internet search tips and tricks; creating Web sites; getting more hits on your blog; computer repair and maintenance; salvaging information from old machines; mastering specific programs for specific purposes—"PowerPoint for high school teachers," for example)

- Cooking (finding, sharing or creating recipes; mastering techniques; shopping for exotic ingredients; making everyday comfort food taste like haute cuisine)

- Decorating (interior design; party themes; shopping for unusual and eclectic objects)

- Exercise (weight loss; aesthetics; sports performance; getting started; sticking with a long-term program)

- Language skills (master or teach a second language; learn just enough of a language to make travel in a foreign country more enjoyable; improve vocabulary; learn better ways to explain concepts; become a better conversationalist)

- Martial arts (basic skills; real-world self-defense; teaching martial arts to kids with special needs)

- Musical instruments (how to tune or repair them; how to buy one new or used; how to teach others to play them; how to restore antique instruments)

- Parenting (dealing with difficult teens; surviving as a single parent; helping mixed-race or mixed-religion families cope; shopping for the best bargains in strollers, cribs and other baby gear)

- Regional interests (reviews of area restaurants; best stores in a variety of categories; how to find the best contractors or doctors or other professionals in your area; shortcuts for commuters)

- Travel (the best places to stay; how to save money while traveling; how to save money for traveling; everything a traveler would want to know about a particular place)

- Video games (winning at specific games or types of games; buying and selling; learning cheat codes; finding rare vintage games; trouble-shooting specific game systems)

You don't have to be the best in the world in any of these areas, or any other areas in which you have an interest. You just have to be more knowledgeable, skilled, or experienced than the person buying your product.

Now, having said that, I don't want you to misinterpret my words and think you can sell products with inaccurate or useless information, or pedestrian tips that your customer could find in a few seconds with a simple Google search.

You must be able to deliver whatever you've promised to deliver, for two big reasons:

1. **Ethics.** If you're taking the customer's money, you have to make a sincere effort to give that customer the best and most useful information you can deliver.

2. **Profit.** A customer who feels burned by your first product will never buy your next product. It's *much* harder to find a new customer than it is to sell a follow-up product to an existing client.

In other words, you must deliver value. But that's true of any job in which you're being compensated. If you work for someone else, you know that your boss will fire you if your work doesn't rise to the value of your compensation, in his judgment. If you work for yourself by creating and selling information products, your customers will fire you if your products don't deliver what they expect for the price they've paid.

How to Create an Information Product in One Day, Even if You Have no Skills or Specialized Knowledge

Let's say you're interested in a particular topic, but don't feel as if you have the knowledge, skill, and experience to produce a valuable information product. You can still make money from your area of interest by creating a *compilation* product.

Maybe you're interested in leadership training, but you know you're at the front end of the learning process. You aren't yet a leader or someone who can train leaders. But you're fascinated by the subject and want to know more.

You can create an information product now—as in, starting today—by making a list of the experts in this area, the people you admire and hope to emulate. Include some people who've written about leadership, as well as people who in your estimation are great leaders in their professions or avocations. Find some big names in the field, but also some people who aren't as well known.

Google them and get their contact information.

Now ask each one if you can conduct an interview for your upcoming project. Successful people love to share their expertise and wisdom with others. Their time is valuable, of course, but you'd be surprised at how accommodating they can be. Make sure to let them know you'll be recording the interview, and that you'll include it in a product you're selling—a book, audio program, newsletter, or whatever it is. You'll want to get their written permission to use this information, or at least an email in which it's clear they understand and agree to participate in your project.

Once you have a handful of these interviews on tape—how many you need depends on the length and quality of the interviews—you can sell them as an audio CD, a series of CDs, or downloadable audio files.

You can also transcribe the interviews (or pay to have them transcribed), edit the transcripts, and sell the collection as a book, manual, or series of downloadable text files.

Or you can do both: Package the audio CDs with the written transcripts and offer it as a multimedia package. If the information and insights contained in the interviews are really good, useful, and not obvious or well known, you have a product that can sell for a premium price--$100, $400, maybe even more.

I created a compilation program called *Speed Experts* (<u>speedexperts .com</u>). I asked 18 different strength coaches to create a 30-day speed-training program. Altogether, the programs comprise more than 800 downloadable pages. It sells for $97 online.

A student of mine, Virgil Aponte, borrowed this idea and did the same thing for improving vertical jump (<u>jumpexperts.net</u>). Another student, Jen Heath, took this concept for fat loss and created <u>thefatlosspros.com</u>.

A Business You Can Run on Autopilot

By the time you finish reading The Millionaire Workout you'll have dozens of ideas for different information products you can create. But, for the purposes of the 21-day coaching program, I want you to think about one particular type of product: an e-book.

An e-book can be as short and simple as a 50-page report sold as a PDF file, or as big and complex as you want to make it, with the caveat that whatever you produce can be downloaded by your customers.

Here's why I think an e-book is the perfect inaugural product:

- **No inventory.** Customers purchase your product and download it to their computers. You can turn a profit from the very first sale, and use your profits for marketing this product or creating new ones.

- **No printing.** If your customers want a printed copy, they'll use their own equipment. That saves you time and money.

- **Nothing to ship.** Fulfillment is automatic—once the customer has paid for and downloaded the product, the transaction is complete. You don't have to worry about buying envelopes, printing mailing labels, and making daily runs to the post office.

- **No limit to your sales.** A digital product can be sold an infinite number of times to as many customers as you can generate. That means there's no limit to the amount of money you can make on a single product, or a line of products.

- **No barrier to entry.** Like I've been saying, anyone can get into the business of producing and selling information products. It's not like getting into Harvard or running for office. Entrepreneurs are self-selected.

- **No need for you to be present.** Once you've created and set up the mechanism for selling the product, it's always on sale. Anyone with a credit card and Internet access can buy it. You can be anywhere, doing anything, and never have to worry about sales and fulfillment.

I hope you're excited about the idea of getting into this business. I'm looking forward to showing you exactly how to do it. First, though, I want to introduce you to the "workout" part of The Millionaire Workout. In the next few chapters, you'll learn how to get in great shape—possibly the best shape of your life—in less time than you ever imagined. In fact, I'm going to show you how to improve your fitness levels dramatically in as little as four minutes a day.

If you're ready, let's get started.

IV

THE FASTEST
WORKOUT IN THE WORLD

I'm going to put it bluntly: I've never seen anyone reach his or her peak potential without regular exercise. I can't tell you exactly why exercise has that effect, although I suspect it has something to do with giving you more energy and helping you feel better about yourself.

If you aren't currently exercising consistently, the 21-day coaching program will show you how easy and rewarding it is. You'll make workouts part of your regular routine, and wonder why you took so long to get into the habit. Why am I so confident? Because my workouts are shorter, simpler, and more effective than any you've seen before.

How to Get Results in a Fraction of the Time

I'm an unwavering optimist in most aspects of life. But I'm also realistic. I know relatively few people have the time, energy, or even the desire to work out an hour or more a day. Even when I was just starting my career as a trainer, way back in 1994, I saw how hectic my clients' lives were. For a lot of them, a one-hour personal-training session three times a week was too big a commitment. They had jobs, families, and time-consuming commutes to get from one to the other. And this was before most of us had email and cell phones.

That's when I decided to try something that was unheard of at the time: I scheduled my clients for 30-minute "express" sessions. Back then, all of gym life was divided into one-hour increments. Fitness classes and personal-training sessions started every hour on the hour. The idea of half-hour workouts was radical enough, but I went beyond that: I didn't want my clients to get half the benefits in half the time. I wanted them to get everything they'd expect from a 60-minute workout.

I also booked the kids I trained at the hospital in 30-minute sessions. For young people suffering with or recovering from serious illnesses and injuries, shorter workouts just made more sense. But, again, I didn't want compromised results.

Later, when I taught physical education at the alternative high school in the Bronx, I had an even bigger challenge: By the time my students got to class, changed into their workout clothes, and gave me enough of their attention to get started, I was lucky if we had 20 minutes left for exercise.

In all three situations, I pushed up the intensity of the workouts. (With the kids in the hospital, "intensity" is of course relative to what they could do safely.) I took out all the time-wasting single-joint exercises like biceps curls and triceps extensions and concentrated on full-body, multi-joint movements. I experimented with work and rest intervals, decreasing the amount of rest between sets or drills. Every aspect of the workouts, every variable, was in play.

Then I came across studies by Izumi Tabata, an exercise scientist in Japan, published in 1996 and '97 in a journal called *Medicine & Science in Sports & Exercise*. Dr. Tabata and his research team experimented with exercise intervals, comparing normal-intensity bouts of work with super-high-intensity bouts. The Tabata protocol featured 20-second bouts of all-out effort with 10-second rest periods. The entire workout, eight of these work-rest intervals, could be completed in four minutes.

The results were extraordinary. Participants in the studies who did the four-minute workouts not only increased their ability to do anaerobic exercise, which is the type of exercise that features all-out efforts like sprints, but also their aerobic capacity. You know that aerobic exercise is the type that's typically done at a steady pace with the idea of developing endurance. If you're going so fast you're out of breath, it's not aerobic, because the aerobic energy system requires your body to use oxygen to generate the energy that keeps you moving. Dr. Tabata and his colleagues showed that anaerobic exercise could be used to increase our aerobic capacity, which was interesting enough, but also that this could be accomplished in less time than anyone had previously imagined.

The one catch is that the Tabata intervals are too intense for most people. But I liked the basic idea so much that I manipulated the variables (incorporating strength training, for example) and came up with a system that was flexible enough for exercisers at any level. So the workouts you do in the 21-day coaching program aren't Tabata intervals, but they're inspired by the same basic ideas. You'll improve your overall fitness levels a maximum amount in minimal time, without ever doing any traditional endurance exercise. The strength training will help you get stronger and leaner, and the workouts are short enough that you squeeze them into any schedule, no matter how hectic.

In case you're wondering, I practice what I preach. I haven't done any "cardio" training for more than six years. All my own workouts feature variations on the high-intensity intervals I prescribe for you and my clients. I'm usually in the shower 15 to 20 minutes after lacing up my sneakers. By my estimation, I save an hour a day with this training system, and believe me, I'd rather spend that time with my wife and daughters than jogging around a track or grinding out sets of biceps curls in a gym.

The Key to Fast and Sustainable Fat Loss

EPOC is one of my favorite acronyms in exercise science. It stands for "excess post-exercise oxygen consumption," which is the key to getting long-lasting fat loss from short-duration workouts. We all know that we burn more calories when we're up and moving than we do when we're sitting around watching TV. Most exercise advice is based on the idea that the only calories that matter are the ones you burn during a workout, when you're exercising, breathing hard, and consuming more oxygen than normal. That's why, traditionally, we've been told that we have to do long, tedious, steady-pace workouts like jogging or cycling if we want to lose fat.

But there's another way to consume oxygen, which in this context is synonymous with burning more calories. If you work really hard, even for a relatively short time, you keep burning calories after your workout is completed. That post-exercise oxygen consumption can be mild and brief if you've done low-intensity exercise. Or it can be big and last a day or two, in the case of a super-intense weight-lifting session done by elite and highly trained athletes.

I can't possibly predict how much EPOC any particular workout can deliver for any individual exerciser. But I can tell you that the higher the intensity of the workout you do, the more EPOC it delivers. That's why high-intensity exercise is so valuable: The biggest benefits accrue after you stop training.

The Myth of the Fat-Burning Zone

Let's clear up one issue before we go any farther: For most of us, burning calories sounds nice, but burning *fat* calories is the real goal. That's where a lot of things get confused, and where a little knowledge can obscure the big picture. If you have it in your mind that the best exercise routine is the one that burns the most fat, you're going to think that endurance exercise (also called "aerobics" or "cardio") is the best choice, since a human body will use more fat for energy during steady, low-intensity exercise. You'll also stay away from strength training and high-intensity interval-type training, since we rely on carbohydrate for energy during anaerobic exercise.

This is basic physiology, and I have no beef with it. What I object to is the idea that the type of energy we use during the exercise itself is the most important consideration. In other words, forget about exercising in the "fat-burning zone." It's a distraction. You ultimately burn more calories, including more fat calories, with anaerobic exercise.

Here's a simplified example:

Let's say you go for an easy jog for 30 minutes during you leave for work in the morning, and let's say you burn 150 calories beyond the calories your body would've used if you'd just stayed in bed for an extra half-hour.

But instead of jogging for 30 minutes, let's say you do one of my Millionaire Workout routines for 12 minutes, and you burn 100 calories more than you would if you'd stayed comfortably horizontal.

As a jogger, you've burned more calories, and probably more fat calories as well. But that advantage disappears when you figure EPOC into the equation. While you're getting that post-workout "afterburn," *you're burning a higher percentage of fat calories* than you would if you hadn't exercised at all, in addition to the fact that *you're burning total calories at a faster pace.*

I'd be lying if I said I could give you a precise calculation of how many calories you'll burn during or after a workout, but I'd also be shocked if you didn't come out ahead by doing my workout for 12 minutes instead of trudging around the block for 30 minutes.

Here's another way to look at it.

If you buy into the idea of a fat-burning zone, then basic science tells us that the slower you go, the higher the percentage of fat you'll use for energy. That means you're burning the highest percentage of fat calories when you're moving the least. In other words, the ideal fat-burning exercise is sleeping. Watching TV would come in a close second.

So let's forget about the fat-burning zone, and tackle a more substantive issue.

One of the best arguments in favor of steady-pace endurance exercise is that you can burn more calories per workout, since you can exercise longer. Common sense tells us that you'll burn more calories jogging for an hour than you will in one of my 12-minute workouts. Even when you add in the calories you'll burn with EPOC, that hour of jogging still comes out ahead.

Why, then, do I recommend shorter, higher-intensity workouts?

One word: results.

Something extraordinary happens when you train using high-intensity exercise. A study at Laval University in Quebec, published in a journal called *Metabolism* back in 1994, showed that high-intensity exercise burned off significantly more body fat than steady-state endurance exercise. We aren't talking about calories burned during exercise here, or whether they came from fat or carbohydrate. We're talking about actual fat that disappeared from actual bodies. The researchers came up with this calculation: Each calorie you burn during high-intensity exercise strips off nine times more fat than a calorie burned during steady-pace exercise.

So to match the results you can get from a 12-minute workout, you'd have to burn off *nine times as many calories* jogging.

If you see the logic of focusing on high-intensity exercise, let's get into some of the specifics of the *Millionaire Workout* routines. **MW**

V

Six-Pack Abs for a Seven-Figure Earner

B efore I tell you more about the *Millionaire Workout* system, I'll tell you what you won't find: biceps curls, triceps kickbacks, leg extensions, or any other exercise that attempts to work your muscles in isolation. You also won't see boring gym staples like the barbell bench press. You can see those in hundreds of workout books, but not this one.

What you will find are a mix of unique exercises that you probably haven't seen before, along with some fun variations on traditional moves. A lot of us thought we'd left behind classic exercises like the pushup the last time we did them in gym class. But those exercises became classics for a reason. They require coordination and work lots of major muscle groups at the same time, rather than attempting to isolate some while overworking others.

And they're almost infinitely versatile. For example, I know more than 100 different ways to do a pushup. That's right, triple-digit variations on what you probably thought was a simple exercise. Start with the basic pushup, with both hands and feet on the floor. You can make it easier with an incline (hands higher than feet), or harder with a decline (feet higher than hands). You can position your hands wider or bring them in closer. You can change it up by putting one or both hands on a medicine ball. You can do a plyometric pushup, in which you push yourself up with so much force that your hands come off the floor. You can do pushups with one foot off the floor, or with both feet on a stability ball, or with your hands on a stability ball, or with your hands on one stability ball and your feet on another. If you're really strong, you can do handstand pushups or even one-armed pushups, like Rocky.

I included a few of those variations in the coaching program, along with many of my favorite full-body exercises. My goal is to help you do the most work in the least amount of time for the biggest impact on your body.

Getting Fit, Four Minutes at a Time

The key to a successful workout program is progression. The fundamental problem with Curves and other facilities that offer 30-minute circuit workouts is that there's no progression—you do the same exercises in the same way every time, without moving on to more challenging routines. These programs are fine for absolute beginners, since they're simple and accessible. Anything that gets sedentary people moving and taking action is great, in my view. But after a few weeks or months of the exact same workouts, you'll hit a plateau.

You won't have to worry about stalling out in the 21-day coaching program. Progression is built into the program three different ways:

• Your exercise time increases

• Your rest periods between exercises decrease

• The exercises themselves become more challenging

After 21 days, you can either create your own workouts, or you can have me continue to coach you in your home with new workouts delivered each month via newsletter. (**Check out the details at ryanlee.com/insider**.)

The workouts are all four minutes long. You'll start with a single four-minute workout and build up to three four-minute workouts performed consecutively. The longest program you'll ever do is 12 minutes.

Each workout features eight exercises. Sometimes it will be eight different exercises that you do once each, but in other workouts you'll repeat one exercise eight times.

However, just because the workouts are short and relatively straightforward, you shouldn't assume they're going to be easy. If the workout calls for you to do pushups for 20 seconds, for example, you need to do as many pushups as possible in those 20 seconds. The deeper you get into the program, and the more your conditioning improves, the more repetitions you should be able to do in each set.

Some of you won't be able to do some of these exercises continuously for the entire time allotted. But even if you have to stop halfway through to catch a breath, it's still important that you keep trying. If the set is supposed to last 20 seconds, you can't stop at 15 seconds and use the extra five seconds for rest before the next exercise. You have to push yourself for the entire 20 seconds.

You'll need a watch or, better yet, a stopwatch to make sure you time the work and rest intervals correctly.

Ideally, you want to do the workouts first thing in the morning, before life gets in the way. Plus, you'll feel a sense of accomplishment when you start your day with an invigorating workout. If you don't already have enough time in your schedule to accommodate that, just set your alarm clock to go off 15 minutes earlier. If even that is a challenge, then start tomorrow by setting your clock back one minute earlier and every day increase by another minute until you're at 15 minutes.

And with that, we're finished with the theories behind my Millionaire Workout routines. Chapter 6 shows you the exercises you'll do, and then (finally!) we'll get into the 21-day coaching program. **MW**

VI

THE EXERCISES

W hen I named this book *The Millionaire Workout*, I started with the assumption that you aren't yet wealthy. But since I want you to become a millionaire—or at least closer to that distinction than you are now—the last thing I want you to do is waste your time or money getting to that point.

You already know that the workouts top out at 12 minutes, so time won't be a factor.

I've also made the workouts as accessible as possible. You can do lots of exercises with no equipment at all—all you need is 10 feet of open space. The other exercises require a pair of dumbbells. It would be better to have an entire set, of course, but you can do the workouts with just one pair.

Dumbbells are cheap. Plain hexagonal dumbbells cost about 50 cents per pound at your local sporting-goods store. A pair of 15-pounders will run about $20.

And that's it—you don't need a $5,000 treadmill or elliptical trainer, nor do you have to clear out space for a complete home gym. There's nothing wrong with having a full set-up at home, but for the 21-day coaching program, you won't need it.

Exercise Categories

I divided the exercises into five categories:

Workout Prep: You'll do these exercises before your workout, to make sure your body is ready for more strenuous and challenging drills.

Total Body: These exercises work all your major muscle groups.

Upper Body: The focus is on the big upper-body muscles in your chest, back, and shoulders. You'll also work your arms with these exercises, but I didn't include any exercises that attempt to isolate your arm muscles.

Lower Body: These exercises work your body's biggest and strongest muscles—those in your hips (including your gluteals) and legs.

Core: You'll work your midsection—abs and lower back—with these exercises.

Anaerobic: These drills are designed to get your heart rate up and elevate your post-workout metabolism.

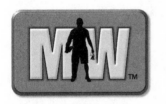 # Workout Prep

4-way neck rotation

1. Start by tilting your head backward and slowly rotating it to the side in one fluid motion.

2. Halfway through the movement, you should have your head titled forward with your chin on your chest.

3. Complete the circle until your head is again tilted backward.

4. Do the designated number of repetitions to that side, then repeat the circles going the other direction. (You can also alternate repetitions, doing a circle to the right, then a circle to the left, until you've done all the reps to each side.)

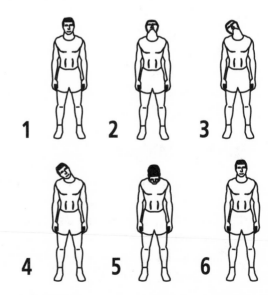

Small Arm Circle Swings

1. Stand holding your arms out to your sides at shoulder height.

2. Rotate your arms forward in small circles for the recommended time.

3. Repeat the arm circles, this time going backward.

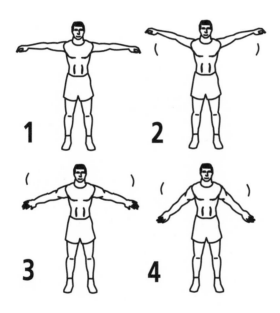

Across Body Arm Swings

1. Stand holding your arms out to your sides at shoulder height.

2. Slowly swing your arms back and forth across the front of your body.

3. Repeat this continuous motion for the recommended time, or until your shoulders feel sufficiently warmed up.

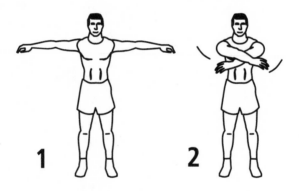

Sideways Leg Swings

1. Stand perpendicular to a wall or some other sturdy object you can use for balance. Place the hand nearest the wall on it.

2. In a smooth and continuous motion, swing the leg farthest from the wall back and forth across the front of your body. Try to hit your full range of motion on the swings without losing your balance. Keep your upper body stable throughout the movement.

3. Do the recommended repetitions, then turn around, place your other hand on the wall, and repeat the set with your other leg.

1   **2**

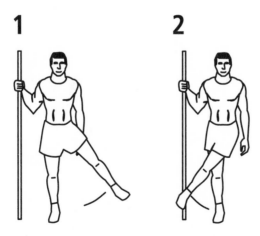

Forward/Backward Leg Swings

1. Start in the same position you used for the sideways leg swings, this time with your feet shoulder width apart. (You can also stand on a small step for this exercise.) Keep your hand near the wall, or even touching it lightly, but try not to depend on it to keep your balance.

2. Swing the leg farthest from the wall forward and back, keeping your upper body perpendicular to the ground. Go for a full range of motion, but don't swing the leg so hard that your upper body moves to compensate.

3. Do the recommended repetitions, then turn around and repeat with the other leg.

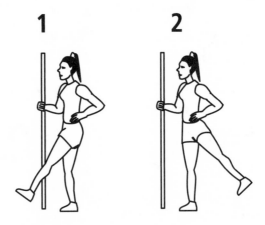

Inchworm

1. Get into pushup position on the ground.

2. "Walk" your feet up toward your hands, allowing your hips to rise up toward the ceiling while keeping your legs as straight as possible.

3. Ideally, you want your feet flat with your palms on the floor at the midpoint of the exercise. Don't force it if you don't have enough flexibility to do that now; just keep working on your range of motion in subsequent workouts.

4. From this position, walk your hands forward until you're once again in a pushup position.

5. Repeat for the designated distance. If you don't have room to go forward more than one rep at a time, reverse your direction on each rep.

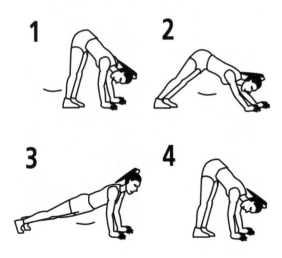

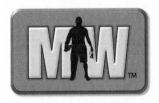 **Total Body**

Dumbbell Curl and Press

1. Stand holding the dumbbells at your sides, using a neutral grip (palms turned toward each other).

2. Curl the dumbbells up toward your shoulders, then continue the movement until the weights are overhead.

3. Keep your midsection tight throughout the movement.

4. Return to the starting position and repeat.

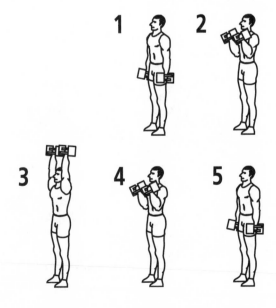

8 Count Bodybuilders

Despite its name, this drill should be fluid, a continuous motion rather than a series of starts and stops. With some practice, you'll be able to do it smoothly.

1. Stand straight with your feet together and hands at your sides.
2. Bend your knees and place your hands on the ground, shoulder-width apart.
3. Thrust your legs back so you're in a pushup position.
4. Lower your chest to the floor, the push back up.
5. Spread your legs, keeping the rest of your body in the pushup position.
6. Pull your legs back together, again without shifting the position of your hips, torso, head, or arms.
7. Bring your knees back in toward your chest.
8. Stand up, then immediately start the next repetition.

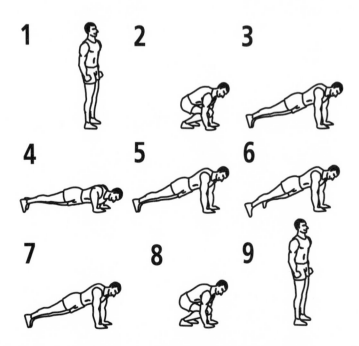

Squat Pull

1. Stand with your feet shoulder-width apart, holding one end of a dumbbell with both hands. Your arms should be straight with the weight between your legs.

2. Squat down until the bottom end of the dumbbell touches the floor. Keep your back in its naturally arched position—don't bend forward at the waist to make the weight reach the floor.

3. Stand up, pulling the dumbbell to your chest.

4. Lower the weight to the starting position and repeat.

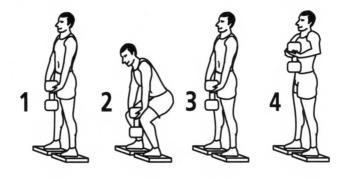

Dynamic Lunge and Curl

1. Stand with your feet hip-width apart, holding the dumbbells at your sides, palms facing each other.

2. Lunge forward with your left leg, and lower your body until your left thigh is parallel to the floor and your right knee nearly touches the floor behind you. Keep your torso upright.

3. Push back to the standing position, curling the dumbbells up toward your shoulder as you do. Twist the dumbbells so your palms are turned upward by the top of the curl.

4. Lower the weights to the starting position at your sides, then lunge forward with your right leg.

5. As you return to the standing position, curl the weights as before. Continue this way, alternating legs on each lunge, until you complete the recommended repetitions.

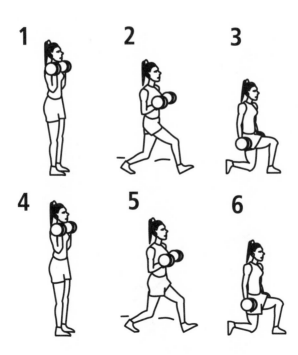

Walking Lunge Curl and Press

1. Stand with dumbbells at your sides, as described for the previous exercise.

2. Lunge forward with your left leg.

3. Instead of pushing back to the starting position, bring your right leg up next to your left. Curl the weights toward your shoulders as you come up, but instead of rotating the weights, keep your wrists and hands in the neutral position.

4. Lunge forward with your right leg. (If you don't have room to do this at home, turn around and lunge the other direction.) Keep the weights up near your shoulders, rather than lowering them.

5. As you bring your left leg up next to your right, press the weights overhead.

6. Bring the dumbbells back down to your sides as you go into your next lunge, repeating the entire sequence for the recommended repetitions.

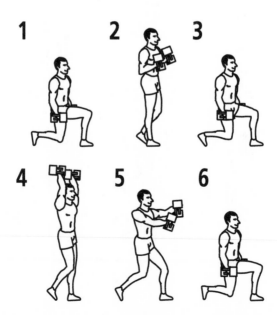

Dumbbell Deadlift Curl and Press

1. Stand holding the dumbbells at your sides, with your feet hip-width apart.

2. Squat down until the dumbbells nearly touch the ground.

3. Stand up as you curl the dumbbells toward your shoulders.

4. Press the dumbbells up over your head.

5. Lower the weights to the starting position and repeat.

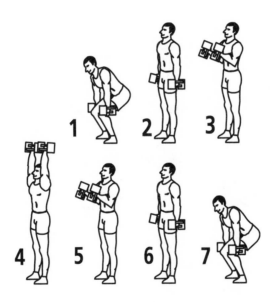

Push Press with Dumbbells

1. Stand with your feet shoulder-width apart, holding the dumbbells at the sides of your shoulders, palms facing out.

2. Lower yourself into a quarter- or half-squat, then quickly reverse your direction and stand up, pushing the dumbbells straight up from your shoulders as you do so. When your legs are straight, the dumbbells should be about one-half to three-quarters of the way up.

3. Lower the weights to the starting position and repeat.

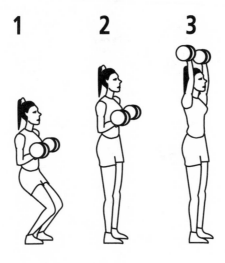

Alternating squat and press

1. Stand holding the dumbbells at the sides of your shoulders, palms facing out.

2. Squat down until your thighs are parallel to the floor, then push yourself back up to the standing position with a powerful, explosive effort.

3. Once you're halfway back to the starting position, push the weights up overhead, using your momentum to drive the weights upward.

4. Lower the weights, then immediately drop down into a squat for the next repetition. Remember, though, that moving quickly and explosively doesn't mean you shouldn't use perfect form and keep control of your body and the dumbbells throughout the movement.

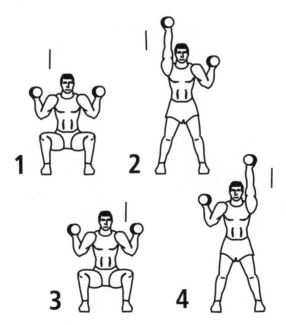

Bicep Curl/Front Raise/Squat

1. Start with your feet shoulder-width apart, holding the dumbbells at your sides with your palms in a neutral position.

2. Curl the dumbbells toward your shoulders.

3. Extend your arms straight out to the front. You want your arms parallel to the floor and perpendicular to your torso.

4. Keep your arms in that position as you squat down until your thighs are parallel to thye floor.

5. Stand, lower the weights to the starting position, and repeat.

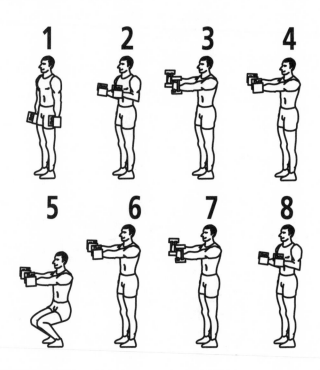

One-Hand Clean and Press

1. Set a dumbbell on the floor. Straddle the dumbbell with your feet shoulder width apart, squat down, and grab it with one hand.

2. In one fluid motion, stand and pull the weight to your shoulder, putting you in the starting position for a shoulder press with a neutral grip.

3. Squat down slightly—you're really just taking a short dip, bending at the knees and hips—then straighten your body as you push the dumbbell overhead.

4. Lower the weight to the floor and repeat. Do all your reps with that arm, then switch and repeat the set with the other arm.

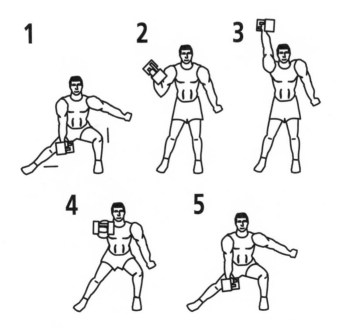

Iron Cross

1. Stand with your feet shoulder-width apart and the dumbbells at your sides. If you have more than one set of dumbbells, use the lightest ones you have. If you don't have any light weights, hold something else in your hands, like water bottles or soup cans.

2. Squat down until your thighs are parallel to the floor. At the same time, raise your arms straight out in front of your torso, parallel to the floor, with your palms facing each other.

3. Hold this position for a moment, then stand while simultaneously moving your arms out to your sides while keeping them parallel to the floor.

4. Lower the weights to your sides and repeat.

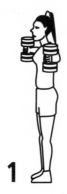

1

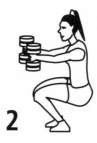

2

Dumbbell Squat and Swing

1. Set two dumbbells side by side on the floor. Straddle the dumb-bells with your feet shoulder width apart, squat down, and grab the weights with your palms facing each other. You want your back flat and eyes looking straight ahead.

2. Swing the dumbbells back, toward the rear of your body.

3. Quickly reverse direction and stand as you pull the dumbbells straight out to chest height.

4. Let the dumbbells swing back between your legs as you squat back down.

5. Immediately reverse the movement as you stand to complete the next repetition. Repeat, making the movements fast and powerful but also smooth and continuous.

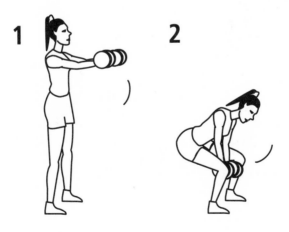

Dumbbell Squat and Rotational Swing

1. Set the dumbbells on the floor, squat down, and grab them, as described for the previous exercise.

2. Stand and swing the dumbbells to your left by rotating your trunk and shoulders.

3. Lower the weights as you squat down and return to the starting position.

4. Repeat to the other side. Alternate repetitions to each side until you've completed the set.

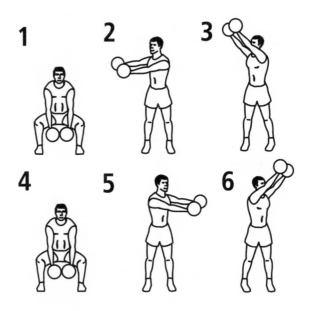

One-Arm Dumbbell Hang Clean

1. Grab a dumbbell in one hand and squat down slightly as you hold the weight between your legs. Keep torso straight but bent forward at the hips slightly.

2. Stand up with a powerful motion, as you would if you were jumping. You don't have to leave the floor, but you come up so explosively that you rise all the way up onto your toes.

3. The momentum from this movement will get the dumbbell moving upward. Keep it in front of and close to your torso, allowing your elbow to bend without using upper-body muscles to force the movement.

4. As you rise up on your toes, shrug your shoulders to keep the weight moving up along your torso. Remember, you aren't consciously pulling with your arm muscles; rather, your arm is a passive lever allowing the weight to move up from the force of your jumping action and the extra pull provided by the shoulder shrug. Your elbow is still above the weight on its way up.

5. When the dumbbell reaches its highest point—roughly the level of your upper chest—rotate your elbow around and underneath the weight.

6. At the same time, dip your hips and flex your knees slightly so the weight lands on the front of your shoulder.

7. Stand straight up, then lower the weight between your legs again as you drop back down to begin the next repetition.

8. Finish all your reps with that arm, then switch arms and repeat the set. Although there are a lot of steps, it's really a fluid motion, and surprisingly natural. Just imagine that you're lifting something heavy with one arm up onto your shoulder.

NOTE: Picture next page

One-Arm Dumbbell Hang Clean

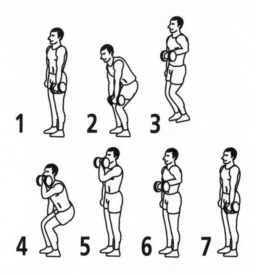

Two-Arm Dumbbell Hang Clean

This is the same exercise as the one previously described, except this time you're using two dumbbells, and landing the weights on both shoulders simultaneously.

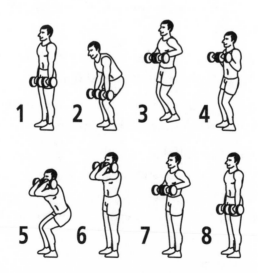

DB Snatch

1. Set up as you did for the one-arm dumbbell clean, holding the dumbbell between your legs as you go into a partial squat.

2. Rise up with a powerful, explosive movement, allowing your momentum to pull the dumbbell up along the front of your torso. As in the dumbbell clean, keep your elbow above the weight.

3. Shrug your shoulders, as you did in the clean. But this time, instead of aiming to land the weight on your shoulder, you want it to go straight up until it's overhead.

4. As the dumbbell ascends past your shoulder, flip your elbow beneath the weight.

5. Dip your hips and bend your knees slightly so you "catch" the weight with your arm straight overhead and elbow locked beneath it.

6. Stand up to complete the repetition.

7. Lower the weight to the starting position, and repeat until you've finished the set. Switch hands and repeat the set.

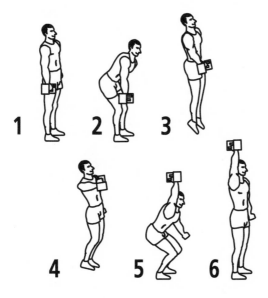

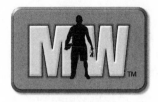 **Upper Body**

Wall Pushup

1. Stand facing a wall, with your feet hip-width apart and your toes approximately two feet out from the wall.

2. Place your hands on the wall, shoulder-width apart or slightly wider.

3. Bend your elbows as you lower your chest toward the wall.

4. Once your elbows are bent about 90 degrees, push back out to the starting position, and repeat.

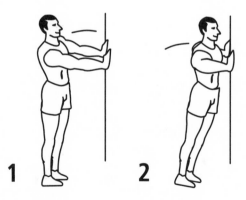

Pushup

1. Get into pushup position with your palms on the floor, shoulder-width apart or slightly wider, and arms straight. Your hands are directly below your nipples, with your fingers pointing straight ahead. Your body is aligned from neck to ankles, and your feet hip-width apart. Your weight rests on your hands and toes.

2. Lower your body until your chest is four to eight inches from the floor, keeping the same alignment.

3. Push back up to the starting position, with your body remaining aligned from neck to ankles. It takes a lot of effort from your mid-body muscles to achieve and maintain perfect form, which is why the pushup doubles as a core exercise.

1

2

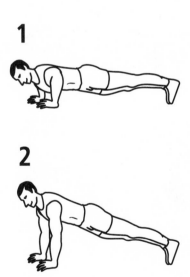

Pushup with Elevated Feet

1. Find a sturdy bench or stool that allows you to place your feet higher than your hands. (The actual height is up to you—you could start low, with a six-inch elevation, and work your way up to 24 inches.) Set your toes on the stool or bench and get into pushup position with your hands on the floor. Remember to keep your midsection tight and maintain a straight line with your body. The only thing that changes is the angle of the line of your body in relation to the floor.

2. Lower your chest toward the floor.

3. Push back up to the starting position and repeat.

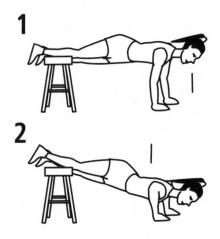

Modified Pushup

1. Get into pushup position with your weight resting on your knees and hands. Your body should form a straight line from your neck to knees.

2. Lower your chest toward the floor.

3. Push back up to the starting position and repeat.

1

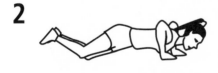

2

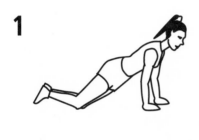

Burpee with Pushup

1. Stand with your feet hip-width apart.

2. Squat down and place your hands on the ground about shoulder-width apart or a little wider.

3. Extend your legs back so your body is in a pushup position.

4. Perform a pushup.

5. Bring your knees back in toward your chest.

6. Stand up, then repeat. As with the eight-count bodybuilders, all the steps should be continuous and fluid.

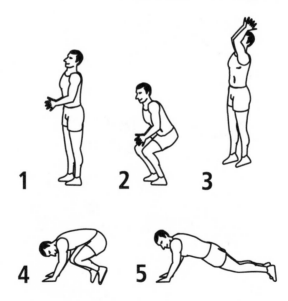

Dive Bomber Pushup

1. Get into pushup position.

2. Instead of lowering your entire body toward the floor, start with your head, followed by your shoulders and hips. It should look like you're diving toward the ground.

3. As your hips get near the floor, push back up to the starting position, achieving the conventional pushup position on the way up. Once you're back in the pushup position, immediately begin the next rep. Your goal is a continuous, flowing motion from one repetition to the next. That said, you're still keeping your neck and trunk aligned, and you don't want your lower back to shift out of its normal, slightly arched position.

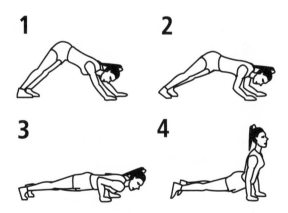

Pushup with Rotation

1. Get into pushup position.
2. Lower your chest toward the floor.
3. Push back up, but as you do, lift your right hand off the floor rotate your body until your right arm is overhead, forming a straight line with your left arm. Your right foot will probably come off the floor as you rotate, so your weight will be balanced on your left hand and the side of your left foot.
4. Reverse the rotation, put your right hand on the floor, and assume the regular pushup position.
5. Perform another pushup, and as you come up lift your left hand off the floor and rotate your body the other direction.
6. Return to the pushup position, and repeat until you've completed all your repetitions on both sides. Focus on keeping your midsection tight and your body aligned.

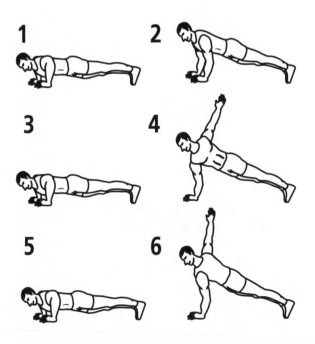

NOTE: More details on this exercise on next page.

Pushup with Rotation (continued)

You can make the exercise more challenging by holding a dumbbell in the hand that rotates upward. In that case, do all your reps to one side before repeating the set with the other hand holding the dumbbell.

For an even bigger challenge, use two hex dumbbells, one for each hand, and alternate sides on each repetition. (If you try this would round-edged dumbbells, you'll quickly realize why I recommend flat-edged hexagonal weights.)

1-Leg Pushup

1. Get into pushup position, and raise one foot a few inches off the floor.

2. Do the recommended repetitions with that foot in the air.

3. For your next set, lift the other foot off the ground. On higher-repetition sets, you can switch feet halfway through the set.

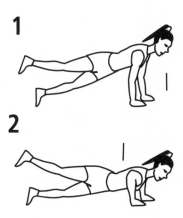

Dumbbell Pushup and Row

1. Place two hex dumbbells on the floor, about shoulder-width apart.

2. Get into pushup position, gripping the dumbbells as if you were trying to crush them. Tighten up your entire body.

3. Push down hand with your right hand while pulling the weight in your left hand up to the side of your torso.

4. Lower the weight slowly, with full control.

5. Perform a pushup.

6. Repeat the row with your right hand, while pushing down hard with your left.

7. Do another pushup, then repeat the entire sequence for the recommended reps.

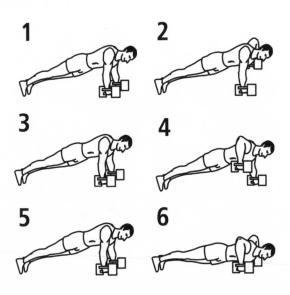

Modified Explosive Pushup

1. Get into the modified-pushup position (knees on the ground) described earlier.

2. Lower your chest toward the floor, then push back up hard enough for your hands to come off the ground as your elbows straighten.

3. Catch your fall with your hands, then immediately lower yourself for the next pushup, and repeat.

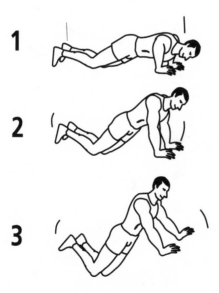

Explosive Pushups

1. Get into pushup position.

2. Lower yourself to the ground, then push back up so powerfully that your hands come off the ground as your elbows straighten.

3. Catch your fall with your hands, then immediately lower yourself for the next pushup, and repeat.

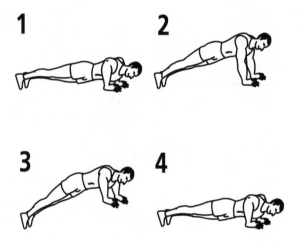

Modified Pull-up

For this one, you'll need some equipment beyond the basic set of dumbbells. The easiest setup is with a barbell on a power rack. Set the barbell at about waist-height on the supports. You can also do this with a chinup bar you buy at a sporting-goods store and put into a doorway. Or you can create your own setup. For a bar, you just need something that's straight, graspable, and strong enough to support your weight. In place of the power rack, you can use chairs, sawhorses, or whatever else you have that's sturdy, stable, and will keep the bar from moving.

1. Lie on your back beneath the bar so that the bar is over your chest. Grab the bar with an overhand grip, your hands about shoulder-width apart. Lift your hips so your body forms a straight line from neck to ankles (same as a pushup), and your weight is supported by your grip on the bar and your heels on the floor.

2. Pull your body up until your chest touches the bar.

3. Lower yourself until your arms are straight, and repeat. Keep your body alignment the same from neck to ankles throughout the movement, just as you would in a pushup.

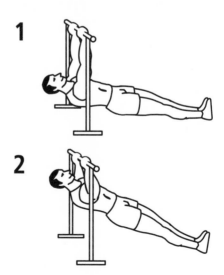

Weighted Pull-up

As with the modified pullup, you can use a real chinning bar or create your own setup. This time, it has to be high enough off the floor for you to hang without your feet touching when your knees are bent. So if you're six feet tall, you want the bar you use to be at least five feet off the floor.

For most of you, your own body weight will provide plenty of resistance. But some will need to add weight. You can do this with a dipping belt, a weight belt with a chain to hold a dumbbell or weight plates while you do pullups or dips; or a weighted vest. (You can find these online at many outlets.) Or you can put the extra iron into a backpack, which you'd wear across your chest (kind of like a Baby Bjorn, a reference you'll get if you have young children).

1

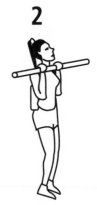

1. Strap on the belt, vest, or pack with the weight you want to add. Grab the bar with an underhand grip and your hands shoulder-width apart, or slightly narrower. (If the chinup bar you're using is too high to reach, use a step to get there, rather than jumping up off the ground.) Hang with your arms fully extended and elbows forward. If you need to, bend your knees and cross your feet behind you.

2

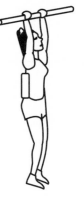

2. Pull your body up until your chin is over the bar.

3. Lower yourself until your arms are straight, and repeat. Keep the movement controlled to minimize momentum and body sway.

Modified Handstand Pushup

1. Stand with your back to the wall you're going to use. Bend forward and set your hands on the floor, fingers pointing away from the wall, and then lift your feet up on the wall until your body is at the preferred angle to the floor. (You want at least a 45-degree angle. The higher you place your feet on the wall, the more of a challenge the exercise will be.)

2. Lower your body as far as you can. (Unlike a regular pushup, your face will get in the way.)

3. Push back up to the starting position, and repeat.

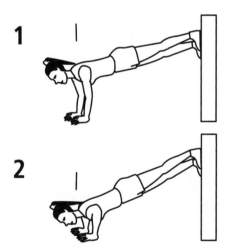

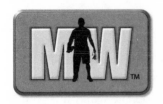 **Lower Body**

Bodyweight Box Squat

1. Set up a box, bench, or chair that's about 18 inches off the floor. Stand with your back to it, your heels about 24 inches away from it. Set your feet shoulder-width apart and parallel to each other, and hold your arms out in front of you.

2. Squat down as if you were going to sit in a chair, with your hips shifting back toward the bench, your upper body leaning forward slightly, and your back in its natural, slightly arched posture. Lower yourself until your butt touches the bench.

3. Rise back to the starting position and repeat. You can make it more challenging by holding your arms at your sides or behind your head.

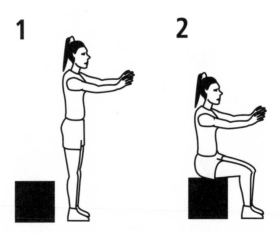

Bodyweight Forward Lunge

1. Stand with your feet together and hip-width apart.

2. Take a long step forward with one foot and lower your body until your back knee comes close to touching the ground. Keep your torso upright.

3. Push back to the starting position, and repeat. Finish all the repetitions with that leg, then repeat the set with the other leg.

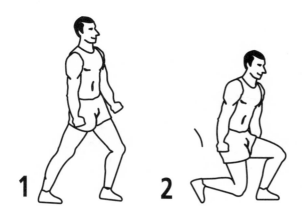

Stationary Lateral Squat

1. Set your feet in a wide stance, perhaps double shoulder-width, and parallel to each other. Hold your hands behind your head.

2. Shift your weight and hips to one side and squat down until that thigh is parallel to the floor. Your hips will drop down behind that foot while your torso leans forward.

3. Push back to the starting position, then repeat to the other side. Alternate lateral squats to each side for the desired repetitions. Make sure that your back stays in its natural posture throughout, and avoid twisting—you should face forward throughout the movement.

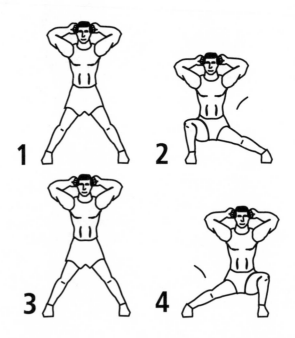

Bodyweight Reverse Lunge

1. Stand with your feet hip-width apart.

2. Lunge back with one foot and lower your body until your rear knee nearly touches the ground and your front knee is bent about 90 degrees. Keep your torso upright throughout the movement.

3. Push back to the starting position. Finish all your reps with that leg, then switch legs and repeat the set.

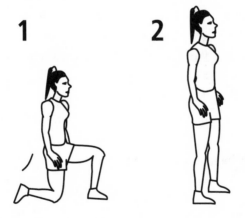

Dumbbell Lunge Crossover

1. Grab a pair of dumbbells (a light pair, if you have more than one), and stand with your feet hip-width apart. Hold the weights out in front of your body.
2. Lunge forward, as described previously, and at the same time swing the dumbbells across your body toward the hip of the leg that's lunging. (Your left hip if you're lunging with your left leg.) Keep your torso and hips facing forward.
3. Push back to the starting position, with the dumbbells once again out in front of your body.
4. Repeat to the opposite side, and then alternate repetitions.

<u>Key safety considerations:</u>
- Step far enough forward that your lower leg is perpendicular to the floor, or close to perpendicular. You don't want your knees to extend past your toes.
- Your back knee should come close to the floor, but not actually touch it. Adding weights and lateral movement to the lunge will change your balance, so you have to careful not to bang your rear knee into the floor.
- Your torso and hips need to remain upright and facing forward, even though your shoulders will turn somewhat as you swing the dumbbells.
- Keep your head in the same position, eyes facing forward.

1　　　　**2**　　　　**3**

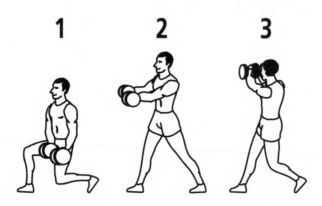

Squat Jump

1. Stand with your feet shoulder-width apart, your trunk flexed forward slightly from your hips, and your back in its naturally arched posture. Your arms should be in the "ready" position, with your elbows bent about 90 degrees and slightly behind your torso.

2. Lower your body until your thighs are parallel to the ground.

3. Leap as high as you can, driving your arms up as you do. Your toes should point straight down toward the floor as they come off the ground.

4. Land on both feet, with your knees soft (slightly bent), and repeat.

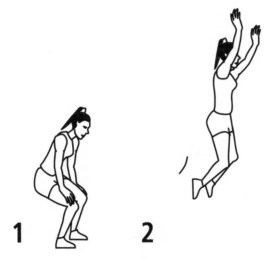

1   **2**

Alternating split squat jump

1. Stand with your feet hip width apart. Step back with your left foot so the toes are roughly 24 inches behind the heel of your right foot. You want the ball of your left foot on the floor, with your right foot flat. Your head and torso are upright and facing forward. Place your hands on your waist.

2. Lower your body until your right thigh is parallel to the floor.

3. Push off hard and jump straight up so both feet leave the floor and your toes are pointed down.

4. Switch feet in midair, so when you land your left foot is forward and your right foot is back.

5. Repeat, alternating legs on each jump.

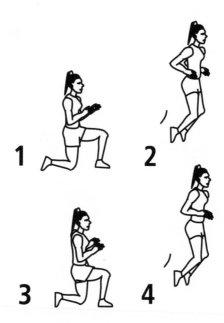

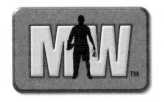 **Core**

Bicycle Crunch

1. Lie on your back on the floor or a bench with your knees bent and feet off the floor. Place your hands behind your head, with your elbows back and out of sight. Your neck should be aligned with your back, leaving a space between your chin and chest.

2. Straighten your right leg.

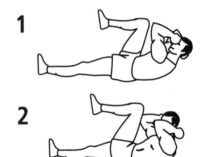

3. Lift your head and shoulders off the floor, keeping your chin and chest pointed toward the ceiling. At the same time, pull your right knee in toward your chest as you straighten your left leg.

4. Straighten your right leg as you lower your shoulders toward the floor.

5. Immediately pull your left leg in toward your chest as you raise your shoulders, being careful to keep your neck and back in the same alignment.

6. Alternate on each repetition until you finish the set.

Alternating Toe Touch

1. Lie on your back on the floor or a bench with your feet up into the air. As before, keep your head and back aligned and a space between your chin and chest.

2. Leading with your chin and chest toward the ceiling, raise your shoulders off the floor or bench as you reach with your right hand toward your left foot.

3. Lower yourself, then reach with your left hand toward your right foot.

4. Alternate sides on each repetition. To increase resistance, hold a medicine ball in your hands, and reach with both hands toward one foot, then the other. To decrease resistance, keep your hands in closer to your torso.

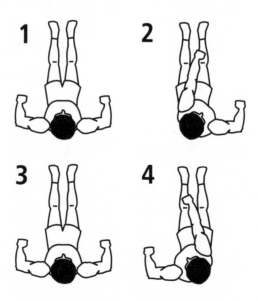

Elevated Prone Hip Extension

1. Stand with your back to a wall, then get into pushup position. Scoot back until you can set your feet up on the wall.

2. Pull one knee in toward your chest, then push it back to the wall.

3. Finish all your reps with that leg, then repeat the set with your other leg.

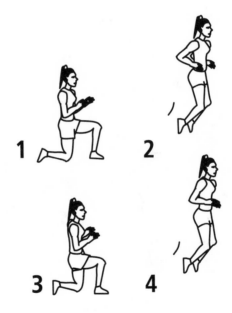

Crunch with straight legs

1. Lie on your back on the floor and lift your legs in the air. Place your hands behind your head or across your chest. Align your neck with your back, as described earlier, leaving space between your chin and chest. Pull your belly button in toward your spine, and flatten your lower back against the floor.

2. Slowly contract your abdominals as you lift your shoulder blades off the floor, leading with your chin and chest toward the ceiling.

3. Instead of lowering yourself immediately, hold this position for several seconds, breathing in and out.

4. Lower yourself and repeat.

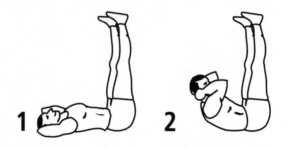

Abdominal Crunch

1. Lie on your back on the floor, with your feet flat on the floor and knees bent. Place your hands behind your ears, as described earlier.

2. Slowly contract your abdominals as you lift your shoulder blades off the floor.

3. Hold at the top of the movement for a few seconds, breathing in and out.

4. Slowly lower yourself and repeat.

1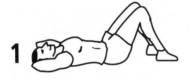

2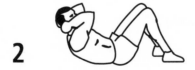

Back extensions

1. Lie facedown on the floor, with your pelvis and toes on the ground and your hands resting lightly under your chin.

2. Contract your back-extensor muscles as you lift your upper torso off the floor, keeping your eyes forward and head and back aligned.

3. Slowly lower yourself and repeat.

1

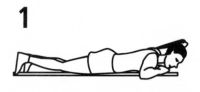

2

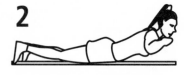

Crunch with 90 degree knees

1. Lie on your back on the floor and lift your legs so your hips and knees are at 90-degree angles. Your thighs will be perpendicular to your torso while your lower legs are parallel. Place your hands behind your ears, as described previously. Pull your belly button in toward your spine, and flatten your lower back against the floor.

2. Slowly contract your abdominals, bringing your shoulder blades off the floor and keeping your head and back aligned, as described previously.

3. Hold at the top of the movement for a few seconds, breathing in and out.

4. Slowly lower yourself and repeat.

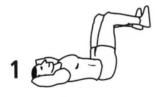

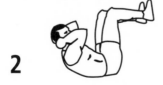

Double Leg Raise

1. Lie on your back on the floor, with your legs straight. You can place your hands at your sides or tuck them beneath the small of your back, with your palms down.

2. Lift your legs until the soles of your feet face the ceiling, keeping your legs straight.

3. Lower your legs until they almost touch the ground.

4. Bend your knees and pull them in toward your chest.

5. Extend your legs again and repeat. If you can't keep your legs off the floor throughout the set, it's okay to let your heels touch in between reps.

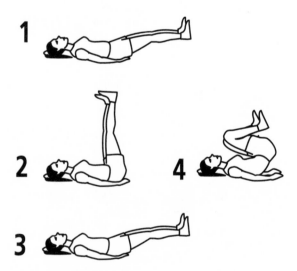

Janda Situp

1. Lie on your back with your feet on the floor and your knees bent. Tighten your glutes and hamstrings, flexing them as hard as you can.

2. Fill your lungs with air, and then raise your chest and shoulders off the floor as you slowly exhale. It should take three to five seconds lift yourself.

3. Return to the starting position and repeat.

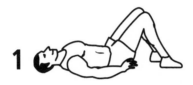

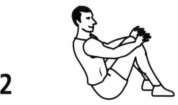

Seated Knee Raises

1. Sit on the end of a chair or bench, with your hands holding the sides of the bench for balance, if you need it. Raise your feet two to three inches off the floor with your legs nearly straight—you want just a slight bend at your knees. Lean back at the hips so your torso is at a 45-degree angle to the floor. Keep your lower back in its naturally arched position, and pull your abdominals in.

2. Pull your knees in toward your chest as you push your chest toward your chest toward your knees.

3. Hold for a few seconds, then slowly lower yourself to the starting position.

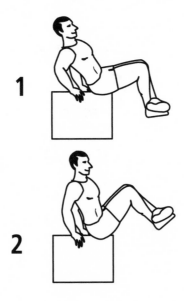

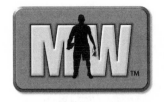 **Anaerobic**

Jumping Jacks

1. Stand with your feet together and arms at your sides.

2. Jump and spread your legs as you raise your arms over your head.

3. Land with your legs wide (perhaps double-shoulder-width apart) and hands touching over your head, then jump back to the starting position and repeat

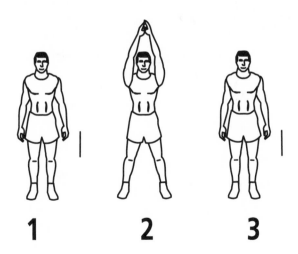

Sprint in Place

1. Stand with your feet hip-width apart.

2. Drive your knees up toward your chest one at a time, pumping your arms as if you were sprinting without going anywhere. You want your feet in contact with the floor for as little time as possible.

1　　　　　　**2**

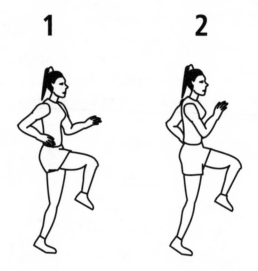

Mountain Climbers

1. Get into pushup position.

2. Drive your knees up toward your chest one at a time, keeping your body parallel to the floor and having your feet in contact with the floor for as little time as possible.

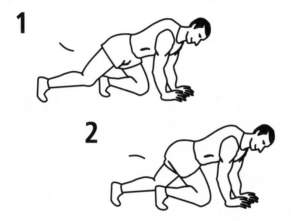

Burpees

1. Stand with your feet hip-width apart and hands at your sides.

2. Jump as high as you can, landing on your hands and feet.

3. Kick your feet back so you're in pushup position.

4. Pull your feet back as fast as you can.

5. Stand and start the next repetition by jumping. Do all the movements as fast and powerfully as you can, minimizing your time in each position.

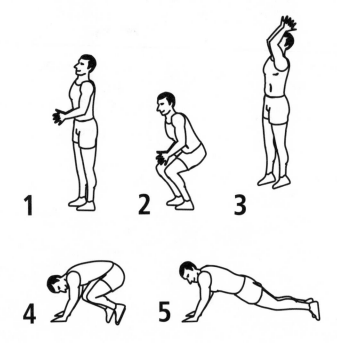

VII

Your 21 Day *Millionaire Workout* Coaching Program

Over the next 21 days, I'll be your personal business consultant, fitness trainer, nutritional guide, and, perhaps most of all, success coach. I'll give you a template that will get you in shape, clean up your diet, and help you launch your new career as an online entrepreneur. The program is based on the same principles I've taught clients who paid me up to $1,000 an hour to teach them.

If you want to see real results, you just have to follow three rules:

- Start on Day 1
- Do everything recommended for each day but no more than that (in other words, don't get ahead of yourself and try to do two days at once)
- Follow the program in order until you finish Day 21

The coaching system depends on progressions to work. Each step you complete laying the groundwork for the next step. Think of it this way: if you were building a house, and tried to construct a frame on a concrete foundation that hadn't yet dried, what would happen? You'd be surprised how many new businesses fail for similar reasons.

The Two Approaches

Chances are you fall into one of two categories.

1. You already know exactly what you'd like to do, the type of product you want to create, and the market you're going to reach.

2. You have no idea what you want to do.

If you're in category #1, you may not be able to complete each step in a single day. It's entirely possible to create a product in 21 days, while simultaneously developing a mailing list and marketing plan, but ultimately it depends on the amount and depth of information you plan to include. Many products can't be written and produced on that timetable. Even if your goal is a shorter, more tightly focused product, you may not be able to work that fast.

That means some of you will need more than a day on some steps. That's okay; just stick to the order and take the time you need to complete each step in the "Get Rich" category. (You'll still follow the 21-day fitness program as written, completing each workout each day. Same with the nutrition guidance—don't hold back on that just because you fall behind on the business plan.)

Conversely, if you already have a product, you won't need an entire day for some of the steps. That's fine, too. You can move ahead, as long as you do all of the steps, and do them in order.

If you're in category #2, you can use the 21-day coaching program as a step-by-step introduction to the principles of product creation and marketing. I'm still going to ask you to "create" a product, but more as an exercise than as a business that you'll have launched by the end of the 21 days. In some parts of the program, the instructions will be more contemplative than actionable—you'll think about what you'd do at this stage, and perform some background research, rather than actually doing it. You could look at it as a practice run. When you're sure of the product you want to create, you can start over at any time and repeat the 21 steps—this time with the goal of launching a real business with real revenue.

Your "Take Action" Checklists

After coaching thousands of people to success, I've found it's best to break large goals into small, easily attainable tasks. That's why I've summarized all your assignments for each day, and put them into checklist form. Simply check off each assignment when you complete it.

If you have to travel or have to take off for any other reason, don't sweat it. Just take the day off. When you get back, continue where you left off.

By the end of the 21 days, you can expect measurable improvements in all three areas. You'll almost certainly be leaner, as measured by your waistline. Many of you will lose weight, which you can measure with a bathroom scale. Some of you may actually have an information product for sale and generating revenue three weeks from now.

Remember, this program is just the beginning of your journey. I have more resources and programs for you at <u>ryanlee.com/insider</u>.

1

DAY ONE

M·W™

M

▼

*Choose your target
market and topic*

*The first step
before you do anything
is to figure out
WHO you will be
selling to*

▲

W

▼

*Ok, you are about to
begin your first workout.
Are you ready?*

*This entire workout
will take you around
10 minutes*

▲

Day One • Get Rich
Choose your target market, topic

Five years ago, I met a baseball coach who had sunk almost $80,000 into filming an instructional video series. He had sold perhaps 50 copies. The problem was painfully obvious—obvious to me, painful to his financial well-being. He spent all that money and invested all that time and effort before he developed a marketing plan.

If you were to disregard everything else I tell you about creating a profitable business, I hope you'll pay attention to this: Your first step, before you do *anything* else, is to identify your audience. Before you build a website, write an ebook, or create a blog, you must know to whom you are selling this product.

I mean, you need to know exactly who your customer is. Who has the interest in this product, and the money to purchase it?

And please don't say "everyone." If you're trying to sell to everyone, you'll end up selling to no one.

There are two ways to narrow down your potential audience in a definitive way: demographics and psychographics.

Demographics:

Here you consider quantifiable characteristics of your customer base: age, gender, race, geographic location, income, religion, political or professional affiliations, or whatever else is a measurable, identifiable trait of your potential audience.

Psychographics:

These characteristics are more subtle. What do they care about? What do they value? What are they afraid of? What pushes their buttons, moves them to action?

Once you know something about the demographic and psychographic characteristics of your target audience, make sure they meet the following three criteria:

1. **They are easy to reach.** You can find them through the magazines they read, their professional affiliations, the websites they visit. A great resource is the SRDS Direct Marketing List Source (**srds.com**). This reference features thousands of mailing lists and gives you a good idea if your market is easy to reach.
2. **They have a passion for the topic.** Golfers are fanatical about their sport. Shoppers love to shop. Parents of school-age children lose sleep worrying about tutors and coaches for their kids, or about whether they're saving enough for college.
3. **They have money and are motivated to spend it.** Just because someone is interested in a subject doesn't mean that person wants to spend money learning more about it.

I've seen marketing advice that suggests it doesn't matter whom you sell to or what you sell, as long as you make your money legally and ethically. (And some don't even pretend to care about the law or ethics.) I disagree. In my experience, you'll not only have a much greater chance for success when you choose a market and topic that interests you, you'll also be happier and more satisfied with the work you've chosen.

Choosing the right market is absolutely critical to your success. Find the audience, serve the audience, and retain the audience—that's the foundation of your financial freedom.

What Will You Sell Them?

Now that you've figured out your target market, you have to determine how you will serve them. It's pretty simple: You will succeed with information products when you know your market well and *solve a problem* for that audience.

That's it.

I've never done exhaustive research, or created complex 30-page business plans with graphs and charts. I just observe my target audience, identify their biggest problems, and solve them.

Maybe it's a frustrated parent whose five-year-old is still wetting the bed. Maybe it's a dedicated golfer who wants to know the inside scoop on the best local courses, or who does the best job custom-fitting clubs, at the best price.

Here are some great resources to explore potential topics:

- listings.ebay.com
- www.ehow.com
- www.mygoals.com

Another tactic is to look through discussion forums to see what issues and questions come up over and over again. When the same questions are asked on multiple discussion boards, especially on multiple threads on a single discussion board, you know there's a problem in search of a product that will solve it.

If you aren't already attuned to message-board culture, here are two places to start:

- groups.google.com
- groups.yahoo.com

So now, on the first day, I'm asking you to make two crucial decisions: what audience you'll serve, and what problem that audience has that your product will solve. Over the next 20 days, you'll learn how to create and market that product.

I can guess what you're thinking: What if I get to Day 7 of the coaching program and realize my Day 1 idea will never work? First, I'd be surprised if the idea you settle on today doesn't have potential. But if you change your mind later, it's still not a problem. Choose something else and go through the process again from the beginning.

Day One • Get Fit

This entire workout will take you about 10 minutes.

Do each exercise for 10 seconds, rest for 20 seconds, then start the next exercise. Continue the cycle of 10 seconds of exercise, followed by 20 seconds of rest, until you've done all eight exercises. This is one "round," and it should take you exactly four minutes.

After you complete the round, rest two minutes (or three minutes, if you feel you need it). Then do a second round.

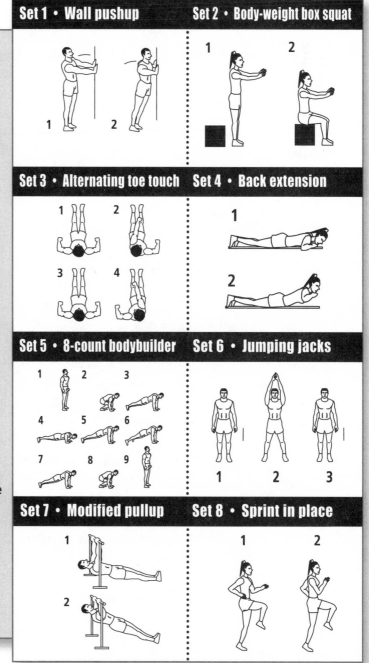

Set 1 • Wall pushup

Set 2 • Body-weight box squat

Set 3 • Alternating toe touch

Set 4 • Back extension

Set 5 • 8-count bodybuilder

Set 6 • Jumping jacks

Set 7 • Modified pullup

Set 8 • Sprint in place

Day One • Eat Right
You are what you... drink?

When a client comes to see me because of a growing waistline, my first recommendation is always this: Cut your intake of any beverage that isn't pure water. Immediately.

Now, I realize this advice isn't exactly original. It appears in just about every diet book and newspaper article about how to lose weight. But you'd never guess that this advice was nearly ubiquitous, judging from the number of people buying larger belts every year.

An average can of soda has the equivalent of about 10 teaspoons of sugar. That's a *lot* of empty calories.

If you're hooked and can't quit cold turkey, start your detox by cutting back to one soda a day. Replace the rest with water. Then cut back to one every two days, then one every four days, and finally just one a week. By that point, your cravings should be finished, and you won't miss the nasty stuff.

Juice isn't much better. Yes, it has some vitamins, but it's still loaded with sugar. The sugar in orange juice might be "natural," meaning it came straight from the oranges that were used to make the juice, with no sugar added. But it's still sugar. And that's in a product that's 100 percent juice. Lots of flavored drinks, from bottled lemonade to Hi-C or Kool-Aid, are designed to look and perhaps even taste like fruit juice, but in reality are just colored water flavored with sugar.

You might think it's okay to drink diet or sugar-free versions of these beverages. And you could be right. Personally, I avoid them. We really don't know if there are any long-term side effects from those artificial sweeteners. In moderation they're probably okay, and even if they aren't they're hard to avoid entirely. But I think large amounts are a bad idea.

So my advice for today is, drink water instead of juice, milk, soda, or anything other beverage with calories. Aim for eight to 10 glasses of water a day. (Wondering if that's enough? You can judge your hydration levels by looking at your urine. It should be clear enough to see through. If it's dark and yellow, drink more water.) You should notice an immediate, positive effect on your weight and energy levels, as well as improved health and well-being in the long term.

Day One • Notes and Action Steps

Get Rich

- Choose your target market. Use resource such as the SRDS Direct Market List Source (srds.com).
- Choose your first topic by exploring online forums found at niche sites and online forums devoted to the subject (you can start with groups.google.com).

Get Fit and Eat Right

- Perform beginner workout
- Drink lots and lots of water, with just one "cheat"—one soda or glass of juice. If you're ahead of me on this and have already given up sweetened drinks, please accept my congratulations. You have a great foundation to build on.

Day One • Notes

_____

_____

_____

_____

_____

_____

_____

2

DAY TWO

M&W

M

▼

Map out all of the
products you could
create for your target
audience

Create at least one
product idea for each
price point category

▲

W

▼

Perform your workout
of the day

Create a strategy to
eat five or six
smaller meals
throughout the day

▲

Day Two • Get Rich
Map Out Your Products

O n Day 1, you chose a target audience and a topic designed to solve a specific problem for the members of that audience. Now the real fun begins: You're going to map out the strategy for your online information-marketing empire.

This is the part most people slip up. I've consulted with some experts who were really well-known in their fields; if you plugged their names into Google, you'd get hundreds of thousands of search-engine hits. But they had no concept of the importance of this step. They thought all they had to do was write a book, sit back, and watch the money roll in. The ones who tried it before they came to me quickly learned that it doesn't work that way.

Instead, *you must create a mix of products at different price points*. I put that in italics so you wouldn't skip over it and miss its significance.

No matter who you are, no matter how famous or brilliant you may be, you can never start with the assumption that it's easy to get rich with one book, or even to generate a modest but sustainable revenue stream. The bestselling authors in publishing history weren't obviously destined for that status. Do you know how much J.K. Rowling got paid for her first Harry Potter book? Fifteen hundred pounds—a couple thousand bucks. And she only got that after the first 12 publishers had turned it down. John Grisham, an unknown lawyer in Mississippi, hand-sold copies of his first published book from the trunk of his car. She's worth a billion now, and he's doing all right. But they're prominent members of a very small minority: authors who get rich from a single product, or type of product.

It doesn't matter if we're talking about fiction or nonfiction. A handful of authors sell most of the books people buy.

The rest of us need a strong backend program.

You've probably heard of the *Rich Dad, Poor Dad* series—hugely successful books, runaway bestsellers. The author, Robert Kiyosaki, started the series to help him market his more expensive backend products, including a financial board game that sells for more than $100.

I'll be blunt about this: I have the same strategy with this coaching program. You've probably noticed that I've mentioned ancillary products throughout the book. If you go to **ryanlee.com/insider**, you'll see products and services that will help you continue the workout program and maximize your income as an online entrepreneur. You'll see a lot more of them as you go on in the book, including endorsements for nutritional products made by Prograde Nutrition (**progradenutrition.com**), a company I helped build.

Does that mean *Millionaire Workout* is part of some shell game, a scam? Hell no. It's a sincere effort to help you achieve physical fitness and financial success, a combination of services my clients have paid thousands of dollars to receive. It's a product that was designed for a specific audience—including you—with the goal of solving specific problems relating to health and wealth. And, yes, it's also part of a line of products. There's no contradiction between the impulse to serve an audience and solve its problems and having a well-thought-out sales strategy including backend products.

Your audience won't hate you for that. They'll thank you for giving them a choice of products at a variety of price points.

Let's get back to the things we addressed on Day 1: identifying your audience, and identifying problems you can solve for that audience. Do you think that any single product will address the entire audience? I don't. People have different learning styles. Some like to read, while others prefer live seminars and hands-on workshops.

Just think of the differences in the way people get to work. Someone who rides a bus or subway might prefer a traditional book. Someone with a long commute in a car might prefer to hear your message via an audio book. And you'll probably have customers who want to read while they're working, but can't open a book or listen to a CD while the boss is watching. But she could get away with reading an e-book, which you'd sell as a downloadable PDF file.

Many customers will purchase their first product from you at the lowest price point you offer. As they become more comfortable with you and your products, they'll gradually move up to more expensive products, programs, and services.

Don't Be Scared of High Prices

Early in my career, I was reluctant to create expensive products. But then I discovered something interesting: The less people paid for my products, the less they valued them. I used to give free consultations. No one would take my advice. I raised my price to $250 an hour, and not only did I have more clients, the clients who paid that amount acted on my advice. I raised my price to $500 an hour, and saw the compliance of my clients double along with the price. Now I charge $1,000 an hour, and let me put it this way: I never have to repeat myself. My clients hear what I say. That kind of money has a way of focusing a client's attention. They hang on every word.

My friend Yanik Silver, a famous and extraordinarily successful Internet marketing specialist, knows the value of high-priced programs. His seminars and coaching programs cost as much as $15,000 per attendee. I can attest that there aren't many empty seats. The longer you're in this business, the more you'll understand that the higher the price you put on your products and services, the more value your clients will perceive. A percentage of your customers won't purchase a product *unless* it's expensive.

Right now, I want you to do something simple:

Make a list of pricing categories for the audience you've identified, using the following chart. Then list the products you could create for that audience in each category. You can do this on your computer in a simple Word document, or with a marker on a whiteboard, or even with a pencil on a sheet of paper. If you want to go high-tech, consider creating a mindmap, which lets you create a visual scheme of all your ideas. (You can find a great program at **mindjet.com**. And no, I don't have a stake in this one. I just like the products.)

Product Categories

Introductory products
$5 to $50
Examples: special reports, e-books, books, CDs, DVDs

Mid-range products
$50 to $100
Examples: software, multi-DVD sets, seminars, tele-seminars, Webinars

Featured products*
$100 to $500
Examples: workshops, multiple-product kits

High-priced products
$500+
Examples: coaching programs, multi-day boot camps
* Over time, the bulk of your sales should come from this category.

I won't go into a lot of detail about these products for two reasons: First, I could probably create an entire book about each one. (I do have a special report listing more product opportunities, which you can download for free at <u>ryanlee.com/insider</u>.) Second, most of you will start with an e-book as your introductory product. As I noted earlier, e-books are ideal for getting your business off the ground. There are no printing costs, and you can fully automate the fulfillment process. Another benefit is that you can update the content of your e-book quickly and easily.

Day Two • Get Fit

Today's workout is similar to Day 1: eight exercises, performed consecutively, working all your major muscle groups. It should take you the same 10 minutes to complete.

But you'll work harder in those 10 minutes by doing longer exercise sets with less rest in between: 15 seconds of exercise, 15 seconds of rest per exercise.

When you've finished the first round of exercises, rest two to three minutes. Then do a second round.

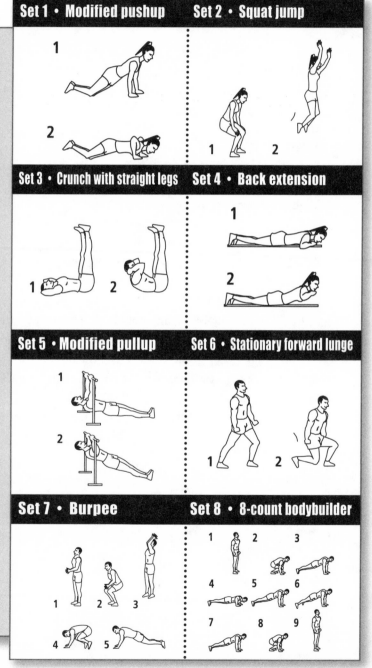

Set 1 • Modified pushup   Set 2 • Squat jump

Set 3 • Crunch with straight legs   Set 4 • Back extension

Set 5 • Modified pullup   Set 6 • Stationary forward lunge

Set 7 • Burpee   Set 8 • 8-count bodybuilder

Day Two • Eat Right
Eat More to Weigh Less

How can eating more be the key to losing weight? It has to do with adaptation.

Your body is quite good at adapting itself to your circumstances. It's a complex system that does everything in its power to keep you alive. So "not dying" is its first objective. Throughout human history, the most preventable cause of death was starvation, which is why your body is very good at sensing impending starvation and reacting to it. It quickly downshifts your metabolism to avoid wasting calories that will come in handy a week or a month from now. If you happen to be shipwrecked on a desert island, this metabolic slowdown comes in handy. But if you try to lose weight by going on a low-calorie diet, or by skipping an occasional meal, your metabolism will react by burning fewer calories, which isn't quite so useful.

It would be nice if your brain could simply tell your body to ignore the sudden reduction in calories—it knows where to find food when you really need it. But it doesn't work that way. Your body goes into emergency mode and hoards the excess calories you've already stored in your fat cells. It also slows down your metabolism, which means that when you go off the diet, the food you eat will be more likely to get stored as fat.

Many dieters end up gaining all their weight back, along with some new weight that they wouldn't have gained if they'd never gone on the diet in the first place. That's why dieting makes so many people fat—it slows down their metabolism, exacerbating the original problem they were trying to fix.

The solution is simple: Eat more often.

Eating frequently will help regulate and boost your metabolism to burn more calories. I highly recommend eating five to six small meals day a day, instead of the typical two or three large meals. Just make sure you're consuming high-quality, nutrient-dense foods, including lean protein, vegetables, and nuts. If you are going to have an energy or protein bar, make sure it's not filled with artificial sweeteners or crap like high-fructose corn syrup.

My favorite on-the-go snack—which, if you've been paying attention, should be no surprise—is one made by my own company: Prograde Cravers (**progradenutrition.com/cravers**). They're organic, taste incredible, and have just 180 calories per serving. I know I'm biased, but I think I'd like them just as much if they were made by a company I didn't help create. Although I confess I might not be so willing to endorse them!

Day Two • Notes and Action Steps

Get Rich

- Map out all of the products you could create to serve the needs of your target audience.
- Make sure to list at least one product for each price point category.

Get Fit and Eat Right

- Perform your workout of the day.
- Create a strategy to eat five or six smaller meals throughout the day, instead of two or three big ones. And promise yourself you'll never skip a meal again.
- Stock up on Prograde Cravers (**progradenutrition.com/cravers**). As long as you know the boss ...

Day Two • Notes

_____

_____

_____

3

DAY THREE

M

▼

*Write a rough draft
of your first
sales letter,
highlighting the
benefits of your
product*

▲

W

▼

*Perform your workout
of the day*

*Schedule your next
food-shopping trip*

▲

Day Three • Get Rich
How to Write Sizzling Sales Copy

Y ou're now at a critical point in the process: Your instinct may be to rush ahead and start creating an outline or rough draft for your product. I understand the urge, and applaud the enthusiasm, but I want you to hold yourself back.

Instead, I want you to write your sales copy.

That's right: *You must write your sales copy before you create your product.*

The purpose of this tool is to sell the product. That's why they call it sales copy, right? But, since there's no product, how can you write something that helps you sell what doesn't yet exist? Isn't there some admonition in folklore against putting the cart before the horse?

Think about what good sales copy does: It describes the product's benefits. It describes the problem it's going to solve for the customer. It tells the customer how it's going to make her life easier, simpler, more effective, or more fun.

When you write your copy *first,* you force yourself to think in terms of the customer: what the customer needs from you (the solution to a problem), as opposed to what you need from the customer (money).

Do this right, and your sales copy becomes the blueprint for the best possible product you can create.

I've written sales copy prior to creating all my products, and my students work the same way. I can't tell you if it would work just as well the other way because I've never tried it. So I confess I have no basis for comparison. I just know I get outstanding results when I write the sales letter first, and, like all my advice in *The Millionaire Workout,* I know it works.

Copywriting 101

Writing strong, persuasive sales copy is a skill. Like all skills, it takes time to master. I'd estimate it takes hundreds of hours of practice to get really good. But since this is an accelerated course, I'm going to give you the basics, pass along a few shortcuts I've learned over the years, and have you write a draft of a sales letter that will leave you with a sound template for your first product.

1. **Headline:** A strong headline draws the reader in, making it the most important component of your sales copy. If you can't come up with a good one, make the first two words "How to ...". The rest of the headline should write itself. You'll almost never go wrong with a "how to" headline.

2. **Create a hook:** Why should anyone buy your product? How will it solve his problem? How is your product better than your competitors'?

3. **Establish benefits:** What does your product do for your customer? Does it make him faster? Happier? Does it help him hit a ball farther, or get a better deal on something he's interested in purchasing? List them all, and describe them in detail.

4. **Use bullet points:** Organize the benefits in a hierarchy—the ones that are most meaningful to the target customer come first—and give each benefit its own bullet point in your sales copy.

5. **Collect testimonials:** Get as many testimonials from satisfied customers as possible. Make sure they are specific and related to the benefits they received. For example, a testimonial that says "this book is great!" is less powerful than "I saved $567.15 on my electricity bill last year using the methods in this book!" These testimonials serve two purposes: They reinforce the benefits you've already promised in bullet points, and establish your ability to deliver those benefits to actual people.

6. **Offer bonuses:** Give free bonuses with your product that add up to a value of at least one to two times the cost of your product. If your product costs $50, give away at least $50 to $100 worth of bonuses. (You'll get ideas for bonuses on Day 6.)

7. **Establish a need for immediate action:** Give people a reason to buy right now. It can be extra bonuses that expire, a limited-time offer, a limited number of products available (or openings, if you're offering a seminar or workshop), or some external factor that creates a sense of urgency (how to take advantage of a tax break that's due to expire, for example).

8. **Never be boring:** Every sentence sizzles. If it isn't exciting, pump it up or take it out.

Shortcuts

Use a software program

As you've noticed, there's a formula for good sales copy. And where there's a formula, there's a software program to help you cut your writing time. These sites will introduce you to programs I like:

<u>saleslettergenerator.com</u>
<u>pushbuttonletter.com</u>
<u>hypnoticwritingwizard.com</u>

Hire a copywriter

You can easily outsource the work. On the low end, you might pay $500 for a three-page sales letter from a solid professional. If you want the best in the business, expect to pay up to $20,000, plus royalties. Two places to find a freelance copywriter:

<u>guru.com</u>
<u>elance.com</u>

Learn to write like a pro

This isn't a shortcut; it's obviously the most time-intensive option since, as I've already noted, it takes hundreds of hours of practice to get really good at writing sales copy. I've been writing my own sales letters for almost 10 years and I'm still learning new and better strategies. But if you're serious about having a long, lucrative career creating and marketing information products, it might make the most sense for you. It's often said copywriting is the world's most valuable skill. No outsider can ever understand the appeal of your products as well as you do, which means you're potentially the best author of your own sales copy.

Some good courses for entry-level copywriters:

dankennedy.com

marketingrebel.com

surefiremarketing.com

For this stage of the coaching program, I want you to sketch out your own sales letter, in your own words. Even if you've decided to hire a copywriter or use a software program, I want you to hold off and try your hand at it first. The goal here isn't to write a perfect letter; it's to introduce you to the process of creating a successful product. Which, as I've said, starts with the sales copy.

Day Three • Get Fit

The time remains the same—just 10 minutes to complete the workout.

But the work sets are more challenging: 20 seconds of exercise, with just 10 seconds of rest.

Set 1 • Jumping jacks

1   2   3

Set 2 • Modified pullup

1

2

Set 3 • Mountain climber

1

2

Set 4 • Feet-elevated pushup

1

2

Set 5 • Sprint in place

1   2

Set 6 • Body-weight squat

1   2

Set 7 • Burpee

1   2   3

4   5

Set 8 • Stationary Reverse Lunge

1   2

Day Three • Eat Right
Shop the Outside Aisles

This simple step takes you away from most of the processed foods in the store. Most supermarkets have their produce (free fruit and vegetables), meat, fish, eggs, and dairy products on the periphery of the store. They do this for a good reason: The highly perishable produce needs to be closest to where it comes in and out of the store. Eggs, milk, and cheese need to be close to the big refrigerators that are kept out of the customers' sight. The butcher who prepares and packages the meat and fish needs room to work, as well as access to the coolers where the sides of beef are stored.

The foods that I call "The Five Deadly C's"—cookies, candy, crackers, cereal, and chips—aren't perishable, so they're sold in the store's middle aisles.

Thus, shopping the store's periphery gets you to most of the healthy items that should form the bulk of your diet—the lean proteins and nutrient-rich fruits and vegetables.

You can't take this practice too far, though. The store's bakery will be on an outside aisle, and you want to avoid that. If the store has a deli, it'll be nearby, and a lot of the food it offers will be just as bad as the Deadly C's.

Meanwhile, you'll find canned and frozen vegetables in the middle aisles, along with canned sardines, tuna, and salmon—all great sources of protein.

The best choices are still on the outside, but you do have to venture into the middle as well. Just don't linger too long there.

More Quick Shopping Tips

1. **Know the store's layout:** Pay attention to where your favorite healthy foods are located, and skip the isles that you know are filled with unhealthy temptations.

2. **Stick to your list:** Don't go to the store and wing it. Make a list, bring the list, and stick to the list.

3. **Don't bring the kids:** If you have children, try to shop for food without them. If that's not an option for you, many supermarkets now offer play areas for your kids, where they'll be supervised and you can shop without their "help." Some stores offer delivery to your home, or will shop for you and bring it right to your car. I've used both those services before. They save time, and you can't ask for a more guaranteed way to stick to your list.

4. **Go *after* you eat:** Never shop when you're hungry. You'll inevitably buy things that aren't on your list, or larger quantities or more easily consumable versions of foods that are on the list. The worst-case scenario: shopping without a list while hungry.

5. **Spend more:** Specialty supermarkets such as Whole Foods (<u>wholefoodsmarket.com</u>) or Wild Oats Marketplace (<u>wildoats.com</u>) are usually more expensive. But if it fits into your budget, these places tend to offer healthier choices (organic produce, grass-fed meats), and a wider variety to choose from.

Day Three • Notes and Action Steps

Get Rich

- Write a rough draft of your first sales letter, highlighting the benefits of your product.

Get Fit and Eat Right

- Perform your workout of the day.
- Schedule your next food-shopping trip. Make a list that focuses on items you'll find on the outside aisles of the store. And plan to go *after* you've eaten.

Day Three • Notes

_____

_____

_____

_____

_____

_____

_____

_____

_____

_____

_____

_____

4

DAY FOUR

M

▼

Chunk your product
into 10 main points,
with two or three
subtopics for each point

Pick the subtopic
you're most
excited about

▲

W

▼

Perform your workout
of the day

Reduce the highly
processed carbs in
your diet, starting
with bread

▲

Day Four • Get Rich
The Five-Step Instant
Product-Creation System

You probably know someone who's working on the Great American Novel. Or the Great American Screenplay. Or some other grand project that he never comes close to completing. Chances are, you've started a book or two, and never finished. Even if you understand that an information product isn't a novel or a major work of nonfiction, it can still seem daunting. That's a lot of blank space to fill.

The best way to tackle any large task is to chunk it down into smaller, more manageable pieces. That's why I came up with this five-step system—it helps me follow a blueprint, allows me to use my time more efficiently, and makes the product-creation process more fun.

The Five-Step System

Let's say you're going to write an e-book for new parents. You've done the research, and determined that the biggest problem new parents face is getting their baby to sleep through the night. Every part of their lives, from their health to their productivity at work, is affected by the baby's unpredictable sleep-wake cycles.

That's the problem your e-book will solve by giving parents effective, real-world strategies, with the goal of getting their babies to sleep through the night in just six weeks.

Step 1: Choose 10 major points your book will address

Major points or topics might include "feedings," "naps," "nighttime rituals," "baths," "room environment," "music," and/or "massage."

Step 2: " Chunk down" each of these points into two or three subtopics

"Feedings" could be broken into three subtopics:
1. Morning feedings
2. Afternoon feedings
3. Evening feedings

Step 3: Write five pages for each subtopic

If each of 10 topics lends itself to three subtopics, and you write five pages on each subtopic, you have a 150-page e-book. If your subtopics don't easily lend themselves to five-page treatments, then go back and reconsider your choice of points and subtopics. Could some of the points be folded into other point? Are some of the subtopics so big that they belong on the original list of 10 points, giving them their own subtopics? This is a great opportunity to hone your product before you've actually started writing it. Just as your sales letter forced you to focus on the benefits of your product, so this part of the process helps you organize the way you'll deliver those benefits.

Step 4: Start with your favorite subtopic

Let's stay with the example of the parenting book. If you love talking about your baby's bath routine, if that's your favorite part of each day, start there. The very first words you write will be about the bathing routine. It doesn't matter that the section on bathing doesn't come first in the book.

This helps you in three very big ways:

First, of course, it's more fun for you, since you get to start with the part of the project that you're most excited about.

Second, you get off to a fast start.

Third, your enthusiasm and passion will set the tone for the rest of the book. When you go back to write the other parts of the e-book, that energy should come through to the reader.

When I started writing *The Millionaire Workout*, the part of the project that most excited me was the 21-day coaching program. So of course I started with that, even though it's the book's seventh chapter.

Step 5: Hire an editor

I've made the mistake of skipping this step, and was embarrassed when I ended up with a product that had grammatical errors. So after your book is written, hire a good editor to check for logic, flow, grammar, and spelling.

For those of you who've started an information product, or feel that you're ready to start one, I'm giving you an aggressive assignment: Starting with Day 5, I want you to write five pages a day, covering an entire subtopic. If you do that each day for the 17 remaining days of the coaching program, you'll have an 85-page e-book.

I don't expect those 85 pages to be polished, or to represent a product that's complete and ready for sale, although you could very well accomplish that. I mostly want you to get the experience of working on a self-imposed deadline (and when you launch a business, almost all your deadlines will be self-imposed), while also showing you how easy it is to complete a project when you have a well-constructed plan.

Beyond e-Books

You can use this chunking system of outlining and organizing for any type of product. Just follow the formula (including the all-important step of starting with your sales letter), and each day you'll get closer to completion. Some products that lend themselves to the formula:

- **DVDs:** Each major point will be a DVD chapter, and every subtopic will be two to three minutes long. Ten topics, each with three subtopics that take an average of two minutes to cover, will give you a 60-minute DVD.

- **Audio CDs:** Same idea. Each major point can be its own audio track. Or you can make each subtopic a separate track.

- **Seminars/workshops:** Extend this formula for a workshop that will last three days, or shorten it to create a one-hour presentation. If your subject material is rich enough, you might be able to build an entire seminar around each of your 10 major points.

Day Four • Get Fit

Today's workout takes about 16 minutes.

That's because you're doing three rounds of the eight exercises, instead of two.

On each exercise, work for 15 seconds, rest for 15 seconds, then move on to the next exercise. Rest two minutes after the first and second rounds.

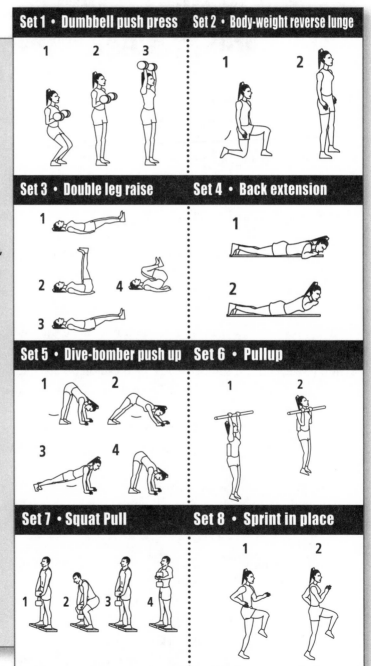

Set 1 • Dumbbell push press

Set 2 • Body-weight reverse lunge

Set 3 • Double leg raise

Set 4 • Back extension

Set 5 • Dive-bomber push up

Set 6 • Pullup

Set 7 • Squat Pull

Set 8 • Sprint in place

Day Four • Eat Right
How to Stop Craving Crappy Carbohydrates Forever

I t's easy to get hooked on sweets and other highly processed carbohydrates. I know, because I was one of the addicts. I slowly weaned myself off the bad carbs, which is why I know you can too.

The problem with these carbs is the lack of nutritional value. They offer calories, but almost no protein or fiber. Without protein and fiber, you won't feel full, and you'll keep eating until you've finished the entire package.

You know about the obvious culprits: soda (which you started weaning yourself from on Day 1), cookies, crackers, cakes, pies. If you're going to have something on this list, make it a special occasion (holiday, birthday), and view it as a "cheat" meal.

Non-obvious culprits include "healthy" subs from sandwich shops and turkey burgers. The problem isn't the turkey in the sandwich or the burger, or the veggies in the sandwich. It's the bread on the top and bottom.

If you must go to McDonald's—and we all know there are times when we're famished and it's the only choice, or the lesser of several bad choices—go ahead and order a burger, but eat it without the bun. If that's too extreme, try it as an open-faced sandwich, and throw away the top half of the bun.

It's easier than you think. Even at barbeques with family or friends, I'll eat a burger with no bun. You get used to it, and everyone else gets used to it as well. Waiters don't miss a beat when I order a burger without a bun at a restaurant.

All that said, if you really love sandwiches, I don't want to induce heart palpitations. I know how you feel. I used to gobble up entire 12-inch submarine at places like Subway and Blimpie.

My first step was simple: go with whole wheat bread instead of the white or Italian. Then I cut back to eating half of the whole-wheat bread. Today, I couldn't imagine eating all that bread with a sandwich.

Your assignment: Take the first small step, and begin cutting back on those bad carbs.

Day Four • Notes and Action Steps

Get Rich

- Chunk your product into 10 main points, with two or three subtopics for each point.
- Pick the subtopic you're most excited about. That's where you'll start writing tomorrow.

Get Fit and Eat Right

- Perform your workout of the day.
- Reduce the highly processed carbohydrates in your diet, starting with bread in sandwiches. If you aren't ready to cut back, at least choose whole wheat instead of white bread, with the understanding that your next step is to cut half the bread.

Day Four • Notes

_____

_____

_____

_____

_____

_____

5

DAY FIVE

M

▼

Choose one method for product creation

You can create a valuable, profitable product in less than one day

▲

W

▼

Write down a nutrition plan for the next day

Purchase nutrition bars, nuts, and other healthy snacks you can keep in your car, at work, and at home

▲

Day Five • Get Rich
Creating Your Product *In Just One Day*

E ven with my five-step product-creation formula, which you learned on Day Four, you might need weeks or even months to write an e-book. But since this is a 21-day program, I want to give you some real insider secrets on how to create products *quickly*.

How quickly? You can create a valuable, profitable product in less than one day—in a matter of hours, in some cases—if you use one or more of these eight shortcuts.

1. Speak it!

Sometimes we all feel as if we're bursting with ideas. We have so much information to offer that it seems to flow out of us like water, once we've opened the spigot. But there's the problem: To create a written document, that information has to flow through our fingertips to a keyboard. Unless you're a professional writer, it's unlikely that your fingers can type as fast as your brain can generate ideas.

But there are ways to get around that handicap. You can simply "speak" your product into a telephone, and a company called iDictate (idictate.com) can turn it into a typed manuscript. If you're really good at multitasking, you can dictate a book during your daily commute.

The company charges between 1.5 and 2 cents per word. Once you sign up for the service, you call the phone number, dictate your information, and let the iDictate typists transcribe what you say. They'll put the transcription into a Word document, and you either clean it up yourself, send it along to an editor, or do both—go over it once, then send it off.

I love technology!

Among your other audio options, you can purchase a digital recorder and have those files transcribed by a freelancer. Or you can go really high-tech, and get a software program like Naturally Speaking (nuance.com), the basic version of which costs about $100. You speak into your computer microphone and let the program will turn your spoken words into text.

2. Interview experts

Another way to create an information product quickly is to interview other experts. For example, if you're creating an e-book for parents that tells them how to help their babies sleep through the night, you can interview experts in the field. Each interview can be a separate chapter:

- A pediatrician discusses possible medical remedies.

- A registered dietitian explains how to manipulate the feeding schedule.

- A veteran nanny reveals tried-and-true methods for helping babies get into a consistent sleep pattern.

Other moms share their sleep strategies. You can find mothers who've worked out sleep schedules in the most trying circumstances—with twins or triplets, for example, or when the family travels to different time zones or the parents work odd hours.

If you want to explore something that's out on the fringes, you could talk to a Feng Shui specialist about how to arrange the baby's nursery for better harmony.

3. Create a compilation

Another great type of information product is a directory, compiling and cataloging information that you have at your fingertips but would be difficult, if not impossible, for an enthusiast to find. By definition these should be opinionated: "The 101 Best Underground Dance Clubs in the U.S.," for example, or "America's Top Family-Friendly Hotels."

There's always a point at which you need to supplement your memory and extensive lists of contacts and resort to pure research and reporting. The good news is that you can hire a freelance researcher to do some of this work for you.

4. Hire a ghostwriter

This is one of the riskiest options. If you hire a competent and experienced ghostwriter, you could end up spending more money than you could to make off the product. A less competent and experienced ghostwriter will give you a product that you may not want to put your name on. That's why I recommend hiring an editor, but suggest handling the actual writing yourself.

5. Purchase rights to an existing product

Many information marketers offer "resell" or "reprint" rights to their products, usually for a one-time fee. Expect to pay at least 10 times the retail price for resell rights, which allow you to make and sell as many copies as you'd like at the full retail price. This can be a winning proposition for both of you. The person who created the product has probably exhausted his sales opportunities, but if you have an audience he hasn't yet reached, you can make a substantial profit.

6. Record a live workshop

You can do a live seminar or workshop on just about any topic (auto repair, cooking, exercise). All you need is a place to hold the workshop, and people to attend. Ideally, the participants will pay you to attend the workshop. But if you're just starting out, you don't even need that. You can get friends and family members to attend. (Just make sure they look like people who're naturally interested in the subject.) Record the entire event (you probably want to hire a professional video crew), put the footage onto a DVD, and you've created an information product in just one day. I've done this with several of my seminars and boot camps, and found it works well all around. Not only is it profitable for me, but the DVDs are popular with those who wanted to attend but were unable to for any number of reasons.

7. Record a teleseminar

A teleseminar—a live conference call in which people listen in and/or ask questions—is a lot cheaper to produce and record than a live workshop. And when it's over, you can sell the audio as a CD or as a downloadable audio file.

I charged $200 for my first teleseminar, which I held four years ago, and sold out all 100 spots, generating $20,000 in revenue. I've been selling a recording of the seminar as a CD set for $199 ever since.

8. Record a webinar

Yet another hybrid product, a webinar is a combination of ideas 6 and 7—a live seminar or workshop you conduct through your computer. You can charge people to view the seminar, then sell the recording as a CD, DVD, or downloadable video file.

A great service called **gotowebinar.com** can automate the entire process for you.

Day Five • Get Fit

This is similar to the Day Four workout—you'll do three rounds of the following eight exercises, working for 15 seconds and resting for 15 seconds before starting the next exercise.

The difference is that some of the exercises are just a bit harder, involving more muscles in each one.

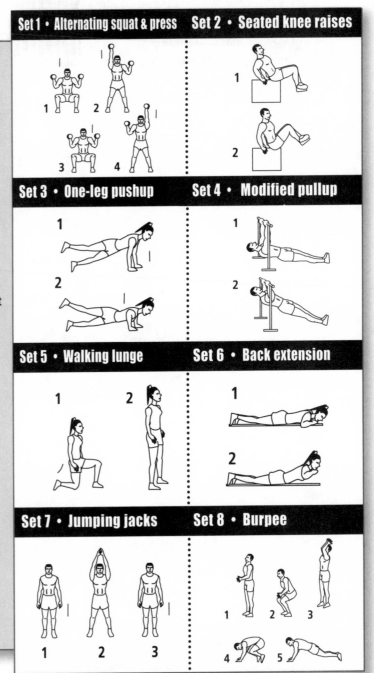

Day Five • Eat Right
Be Aware of Your Nutritional Surroundings

Y ou've probably heard this maxim: "If you fail to plan, then you plan to fail." It's a great motto for any type of business venture, but it's also one of the keys to cleaning up your diet.

You probably have some written schedule of your business day, or at least have an idea of where you're going to be at any given time. That's your starting point. Now, think of how your workday schedule affects your eating schedule:

When do you eat your main meal (lunch, if you work a typical schedule)?

- When do you feel hungry, and start looking around for a snack?

- Where will you be during those times? At your desk? In meetings? In your car?

- If you can't eat at your regular times, when will you be able to eat?

- How much time will you have to eat?

- What food will you have access to? Will you be at a business lunch? Near a deli or company cafeteria? Will there be vending machines when you're ready for a snack?

You can see where I'm going with this. A healthy diet is, by necessity, a well-planned diet. You'd never go into a meeting at which you're expected to make a presentation without knowing what equipment and materials you need to bring. You'd have your laptop charged and ready, and also bring your power cord just in case the meeting runs long. You'd have all the photocopies you needed for each attendee, nicely collated and packaged, along with one or two extras in case a VP decides to drop in.

So it is with your diet. If you don't know where you're going to be at 3 p.m., when your stomach starts grumbling for a little sustenance to hold you over until dinner, you need to prepare for that. It's easier than it sounds. Your briefcase or purse can hold a nutrition bar, a handful of natural almonds in a zip-lock bag, or even a couple of hard-boiled eggs. Personally, I always keep a box of Prograde Cravers (**prograde-nutrition.com/cravers**) in my car, another one at my office, and yet another at my house. Sure, it's easy to do when you own the company that makes the bars, but there are lots of ways for you to stock up and stash away your favorite snacks. If you see nuts on sale, for example, you can buy multiple cans or bags of them, and keep one in each place where you might be when you need a snack. All these tactics help you avoid that late-morning or mid-afternoon rush to the vending machine, or to the box of cookies brought in by one of your coworkers.

But your biggest challenge is to manage the main workday meal. If you're going to a business lunch, you can choose or suggest a place where you know you can find a healthy meal. If you're going to be deskbound, you can stash a frozen meal in the company refrigerator. If you know you'll be in your car driving to your next meeting at lunchtime, you can bring along a sandwich or something else you can eat in the car.

There's almost always a way to eat healthy, but only if you make a plan and follow through with it.

Special Events and Holidays

These take a bit more planning and strategic preparation. Let's say you're going to your Aunt Betty's house for a holiday dinner. You know she'll have lots of hors d'oeuvres—fried chicken wings, cheese and crackers, miniature hot dogs wrapped in pastry shells. It's all stuff you love and find hard to resist.

So you make a plan: You'll have a Prograde Craver and two glasses of water right before you leave. By the time you get there, you won't feel so hungry that you tear into the finger food like a mad lunatic. In fact, you might not feel hungry at all, and only eat something to be polite. The middle ground is fine too: You feel moderately hungry, eat one or two of your favorite treats, and leave it at that. Treats are fine, as long as you limit them to special occasions, and most of all limit the amount of them you have on those occasions. It's all part of being aware of your nutritional surroundings, formulating a plan, and then sticking with the plan without losing control.

Day Five • Notes and Action Steps

Get Rich

- Choose one method for product creation (dictate an e-book, make a list of people to interview, find a product you can obtain the rights to sell, etc.)

Get Fit and Eat Right

- Perform your workout of the day.
- Write down a nutrition plan for the next day.
- Purchase nutrition bars, nuts, and other healthy snacks and meal options that you can keep in your car, at work, and at home.

Day Five • Notes

_____

_____

_____

_____

_____

_____

_____

6

DAY SIX

M

▼

Discover how to double or triple your product value - instantly

▲

W

▼

Perform your workout of the day

Begin to add more fiber to your diet, with the goal of reaching 30 grams per day

▲

Day Six • Get Rich
How to Double or Triple the Value of Your Product — Instantly

N o matter how original, appealing, or well-executed your product is, your sales will suffer if you don't create a good offer to your customers. A good product without an equally appealing offer means you leave money on the table—sometimes a lot of money. Your goal is to create an offer so irresistible that your customers say to themselves, "I'd be crazy to say no."

People will make a purchase based on two calculations: how much value they expect to receive, weighed against the amount of risk they believe they're taking.

Today's coaching session will focus on increasing the perceived value of your product. (Reducing perceived risk is tomorrow's focus.) Since this is the accelerated 21-day course, I'm going to skip the theories of consumer psychology and go straight to my favorite and most successful methods for increasing the value of your products in the eyes of your customers.

Packages and Combinations

If you were looking to purchase a product similar to the one you're offering your customers, which would be more appealing: a single e-book, or a set of three e-books? It's not an idle question. One of the best ways to increase the perceived value of a product is to break it up into components that can be sold as a set. Certainly, you can't do this if your product is an e-book that's only 100 pages long; splitting it into two 50-page e-books does nothing to improve its perceived value to your customers. But if your product is long and technically complex, your customer might prefer to receive it as a set, rather than as one potentially unwieldy volume. And you can sell two 100-page e-books, or two 60-minute DVDs, for more than you could charge for the same material in a single e-book or DVD.

Here's a random example:

If you wanted to read J.R.R. Tolkien's *Lord of the Rings*, would you rather have a single book that's 1,200 pages long, or three books that average 400 pages? Even if Tolkien hadn't written the story as a trilogy, you would probably wish that he had. The most avid reader might hesitate before purchasing a 1,200-page book; buying three 400-page books, even at triple the cost of a single volume, is inherently more appealing and less intimidating.

I did this with my programs at <u>speedexperts.com</u>. Instead of offering a monstrous 600-page e-book, I sold it as 18 different programs bundled together for the price of one. One e-book would be tough to sell for $99, but when I offer 18 for $99, the offer is becomes irresistible.

You can also package complimentary products together and offer them at a lower price than they'd cost if sold separately. You don't have to use two of your own products; you can look for other authors in your field who might be interested in a one-time partnership.

You're only limited by your ingenuity and imagination. You might find products that are in the public domain—that is, not covered by copyright laws—and offer them as part of a package with your own creations. The key is to raise the perceived value of your product or package of products without increasing the cost of producing or releasing the product. That allows you to charge more, or to keep the price the same and sell more.

How to Create Knockout Bonuses that Boost Your Sales Dramatically

Another way to increase perceived value is to offer bonus products. Almost every company or individual that sells directly to consumers uses bonuses. I do it, and I recommend that you do as well. I'll typically offer at least one DVD, e-book, or downloadable audio interview.

A good bonus fits these criteria:

- It must have a high perceived value to your customers, either because of the content or the format. Offering someone a CD or DVD, in addition to the product you want them to purchase, will always seem like a good deal.

- The product must offer something that's either exclusive or, at minimum, hard to find.

- The total value of the bonuses you offer should at least double the price of your initial product. For example, if you're selling a $30 e-book, the bonuses should have a total value of at least $60.

Your goal is to offer a bonus that *presents a perfect complement* to the original product. The bonus should be so appealing that your customers would be tempted to buy the product just to get their hands on the bonus offer.

For example, if your product is an e-book called "How to Make a Living Installing Home Theaters," a perfect bonus would be an exclusive directory of wholesalers that will sell home-theater equipment to contractors for 70 percent less than the retail price. Just one purchase from a wholesaler could be worth thousands of dollars to your customer. Thus, you have the perfect bonus: The directory will have a high perceived value, and mesh perfectly with the subject of your e-book.

That said, I want to throw out a word of caution: Don't go overboard with the claimed value of your bonuses. If you're selling a $30 e-book, don't try to convince your customers that the bonus CDs or audio downloads are worth $5,000. It sounds too good to be true, and your customers won't trust you.

Some more bonus ideas:

- **Audio interview with an expert or author,** discussing a subject that touches on the subject of your e-book

- **Directory of resources** (wholesalers, experts, places to find consumers of a particular product)

- **Your personal Rolodex**—all or most of your personal contacts in your industry (including names and emails)—which will help your customers jump-start their careers in your field

- **Software** that complements the product

- **Access to a private membership site** that offers specialized information and access to people in your field

- **Free telephone consultation with you,** usually 15 or 30 minutes (don't worry about an overwhelming time commitment; surprisingly few customers will actually take you up on this offer)

- **Free access** to a private teleseminar or webinar

- **Downloadable video clips** showing step-by-step examples of how to use the information in your product

- **e-books and downloadable reports** that increase your customer's knowledge without duplicating information that's already in your product

Day Six • Get Fit

In today's workout, you'll go back to working for 20 seconds on each exercise, followed by 10 seconds of rest. Do two rounds of exercises.

When it's a one-arm exercise, switch hands at the 10 seconds mark.

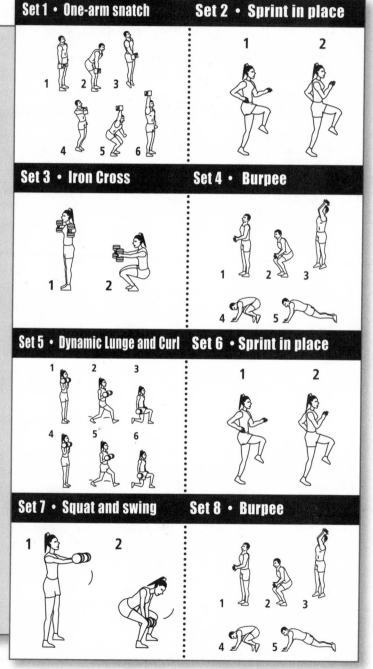

Set 1 • One-arm snatch

Set 2 • Sprint in place

Set 3 • Iron Cross

Set 4 • Burpee

Set 5 • Dynamic Lunge and Curl

Set 6 • Sprint in place

Set 7 • Squat and swing

Set 8 • Burpee

Day Six • Eat Right
It's Time to Bulk Up Your Nutrition

I t's hard to keep up with the all the benefits associated with dietary fiber: lower cholesterol, reduced risk of heart disease, improved absorption of minerals and other nutrients during digestion … the list could go on and on.

Fiber slows down the digestion process, which not only helps you control your appetite and cravings, but also helps control blood sugar, which is important when you're trying to control your weight and limit the amount of fat your body stores.

You should aim for about 30 grams of dietary fiber each day. It sounds easy, but the average American gets less than half that much. And very few foods are rich in both fiber and high-quality protein (the Eat Right target for Day Seven). For example, eggs and chicken breasts have no fiber at all. So your challenge is to include as many fiber-rich foods in your diet as possible—those that deliver at least 2 grams of fiber per serving—without sacrificing any of that high-quality protein.

Here are 15 fiber-rich foods. You'll often see them included in weight-loss plans, since the fiber helps you feel more full, delaying hunger from one meal to the next. They're also nutrient-dense, meaning they offer a lot of vitamins and minerals with relatively few total calories.

Food	Dietary Fiber (grams)	Calories
Navy Beans, cooked, 1/2cup	9.5	128
Bran (ready-to-eat cereal), 1/2cup	8.8	78
Kidney beans, 1/2cup	8.2	109
Split peas, _ cup	8.1	116
Lentils, 1/2cup	7.8	115
Black beans, 1/2cup	7.5	114
Pinto beans, _cup	7.7	122
Lima beans, _ cup	6.6	108
Artichoke, 1 whole	6.5	60
White beans, 1/2cup	6.3	154
Chickpeas, _cup	6.2	135
Rye crackers, 2 wafers	5.0	74
Sweet potato with peel, 1 whole	4.8	131
Green peas, 1/2cup	4.4	67
Mixed vegetables, 1/2cup	4.0	59

Day Six • Notes and Action Steps

Get Rich

- Find one product with resell rights you can purchase.
- Contact one person you would like to interview, with the idea of giving away a CD or download of the interview as a bonus.

Get Fit and Eat Right

- Perform your workout of the day.
- Begin to add more fiber to your diet, with the goal of reaching 30 grams per day.

Day Six • Notes

_____

_____

_____

_____

_____

_____

_____

_____

7

DAY SEVEN

M

Create a risk-free
guarantee for your
product

Begin to gather
at least five
testimonials

W

Perform your workout
of the day

Include more sources
of lean protein in
your daily diet

Day Seven • Get Rich
How to Double Your Sales by Reducing Your Customers' Perceived Risk

As I told you yesterday, people will make a purchase based on two calculations: *how much value they expect to receive, weighed against the amount of risk they believe they're taking.*

Day Six focused on increasing value to the customer. Now it's time to learn how to decrease a customer's risk—and in the process increase your sales.

Offer Powerful Guarantees

An information product requires the strongest and longest-lasting guarantee possible. In my experience, this guarantee translates directly to bigger sales and a longer life for your product. You might be hesitant to offering a guarantee, for fear your customers will use the information in your product and demand their money back anyway. Some will, but I can assure you it's only a small percentage. Few people are inherently unethical. If you make a sincere effort to create a useful product that delivers what it promises to your customers, very few will ask for a refund.

The increased sales generated by a strong guarantee will more than make up for the handful of customers who abuse it. Furthermore, the longer the refund applies, the better your sales … and the fewer requests for refunds you'll receive.

Aim for at least a 60-day refund policy, with no questions asked. Don't just promise something bland and vague, like "money-back guarantee." Make it stronger:

★ ★ ★ **100 Percent Money-Back Guarantee!** ★ ★ ★

We are so confident this product works, if your child is not
sleeping through the night after six weeks,
you can return this program and receive every penny back.
No questions asked.

The Keys to Terrific Testimonials

People are skeptical, and it's hard to blame them. That's why you need to show potential clients that your product delivers the promised benefits. The best way to do that is with testimonials.

I know it seems strange for me to tell you to get testimonials for a product that only exists in your mind, and in the marketing plan you're creating. What I want you to do here is list five potential sources of testimonials. Don't just list five friends or contacts. Throw a wider net. Who's the top expert in the area covered by your information product? Do you know this person? If not, how would you make contact with her?

Now, think of someone you know or have heard about who's had a disappointing or even disastrous experience in this area. How would you get this person to try your system?

Your goal here is to create a blueprint for acquiring testimonials that appeal to a variety of readers and evoke a range of emotions. Some people like to have an expert's opinion. Some want to know that other people in their specific circumstances have used this product, and that it was effective for them. Others are most concerned about safety.

Remember, you set out to create a product that solves a problem. Testimonials are your best chance to show your customers that your product will solve their problem. They also give you the opportunity to show that the product passes muster with an expert, that it's safe, and that it's used by people the customer can identify with on a personal level.

Show Me the Proof

You now have two ways to reduce a customer's perceived risk: an iron-clad money-back guarantee, and testimonials to the product's effectiveness and safety from a variety of sources. Now it's time for the final risk-reduction element:

Proof.

That's right: You need to show your customers actual proof that your program works.

Case studies work best. Pick a handful of people or clients and have them use your product or go through your program. Record their results, and present them as case studies. Remember that these are different from testimonials. You aren't offering opinions about your product here; you're offering proof that the product delivers on its promise.

Sometimes that proof is easy to present. If you're offering a weight-loss program, you can show before-and-after photos, along with charts documenting changes in weight and girth. If you're teaching people how to make more money, you can show screen shots of bank and/or merchant accounts. Black out the actual account numbers, but show the changes in income, wealth, or whatever your product promises to increase. If your product is about shopping for discounts on fashion items and accessories, show a customer decked out in a killer ensemble, and show the price tags documenting the cost of these clothes, vs. similar styles from top design houses that would cost many times more.

If you need to show someone using your program in a video format, you can use a product called Camtasia, available at **techsmith.com**.

Payment Options

One final way to reduce risk is to offer a variety of ways to pay for your product. Some examples:

"Low, monthly payments." These can be spread over a specific period of time, so a $200 product can be purchased in 10 $20 installments, rather than in a more intimidating lump sum.

"Try before you buy." Customers can try your product for free before you begin to bill them. Depending on the product, you could offer a free one-week or even one-month trial before the first payment is due.

"If it doesn't work, it's free." This is a risky but potentially effective option. You're giving the product to customers, and they're only obliged to pay you after they use your product and achieve results.

"Name the price." Tell customers to pay you what they think the product is worth. This option puts even more risk on you, meaning less risk for your customers.

Day Seven • Get Fit

You're back to 15 seconds of exercise and 15 seconds of rest.

Do three rounds of the exercises.

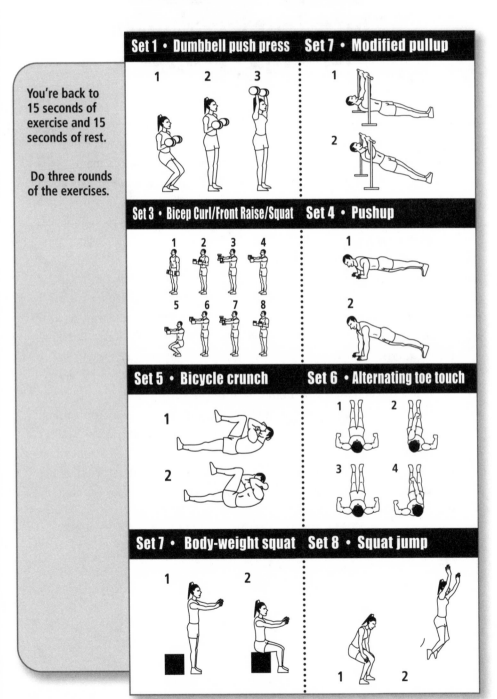

Set 1 • Dumbbell push press

1 2 3

Set 7 • Modified pullup

1

2

Set 3 • Bicep Curl/Front Raise/Squat

1 2 3 4

5 6 7 8

Set 4 • Pushup

1

2

Set 5 • Bicycle crunch

1

2

Set 6 • Alternating toe touch

1 2

3 4

Set 7 • Body-weight squat

1 2

Set 8 • Squat jump

1 2

Day Seven • Eat Right
Stoke Your Metabolism
with Lean Protein

P rotein works like fiber in one respect: It helps you feel full for a longer time between meals. But it does a lot more. Its main role is to give your body the building blocks of muscle tissue. Workouts break down the protein in your muscles, and the protein in your meals builds them back up. The best protein sources include chicken breast, turkey breast, nonfat cottage cheese, lean ground beef, kidney beans, tuna packed in water, skim milk, eggs, and low-fat yogurt.

Until recently, protein's role in weight management was dismissed by nutritionists and researchers. The theory was that "a calorie's a calorie," meaning that your body reacts to all calories in the exact same way, regardless of whether they come from protein, fat, or carbohydrate. But now most experts acknowledge that it's not really that simple. Protein has a higher "thermic effect" than other foods, meaning that it takes more energy to digest protein than it does to digest fat or carbohydrate.

Thus, protein helps you control your weight in two ways: You eat less total food, since protein makes you feel fuller, and you burn more calories during digestion. And, since protein helps you build more muscle when you work out, and the additional muscle increases your metabolism following workouts, you could argue that protein aids weight control in yet another way.

Day Seven • Notes and Action Steps

Get Rich

- Create a risk-free guarantee for your product.
- Begin to gather at least five testimonials demonstrating how your product or system works and delivers results.

Get Fit and Eat Right

- Perform your workout of the day.
- Include more sources of lean protein in your daily diet.

Day Seven • Notes

_____

_____

_____

_____

_____

_____

_____

_____

_____

_____

_____

8

DAY EIGHT

M▼W

M

▼

Jot down a list of at
least 10 different
domain names you like

Register all of them,
or as many as you
can afford

▲

W

▼

Perform your workout
of the day

Schedule one cheat
meal into
your week

▲

Day Eight • Get Rich
Become an Internet
Real Estate Tycoon

Five years ago, I met a baseball coach who had sunk almost $80,000 into filming an instructional video series. He had sold perhaps 50 copies. The problem was painfully obvious—obvious to me, painful to his financial well-being. He spent all that money and invested all that time and effort before he developed a marketing plan.

Domain names cost about $10 to purchase for a year, and $10 to renew each year. It's the cheapest real estate you'll ever own, and potentially the most lucrative.

If you currently have no domain name, it's time to get one, or possibly more. Millions are registered each year, and most of the common words and names have already been claimed. You have three basic strategies for choosing one.

Descriptive

If your e-book is called "The Six-Week Guide to Having Your Baby Sleep Through the Night," you could use a domain name like <u>babysleepguide.com</u> or <u>thesixweeksleepguide.com</u>.

Titular

You can also choose a domain name that will mimic the title of the book. For example, for The Millionaire Workout, my domain name is <u>millionaireworkout.com</u>.

Branded

A third choice is to pick a name that is either made up or has no real relationship to your products. The best-known examples are <u>google.com</u> (search engine), <u>amazon.com</u> (online retailer), and <u>monster.com</u> (job search).

I believe the best option is to create a combination of a title and branded word or phrase.

Millionaire Workout is a phrase that was easily branded as my own. But if I called this book *The 21-Day Success Guide,* and promoted it with 21daysuccessguide.com, it wouldn't work. It's not a catchy or memorable title or domain name, and it's easily confused with other products and programs. Thus, it's a weak brand.

Seven Ways to Find a Great Domain Name

1. Whenever possible, go with a *.com extension as your first option. If the dot-come version of the domain you've selected is taken, don't automatically settle for *.net, *.biz, or the other alternatives. Your customers will always expect you to have *.com. That's what they'll type first if they don't have a link to click through to your site. So if your first choice of *.com is taken, keep searching until you find one that isn't taken.

2. Make sure it's easy to spell. Take it for a test drive before you buy it. Say the domain name to friends and family, and ask them how they think it's spelled. If you've made a good choice, they'll get it right on the first try.

3. Avoid using words that have multiple spellings ("2," "to," "too," "two").

4. The shorter your domain name, the better.

5. Avoid words that call to mind bigger brands and trademarked words. For example, eBay doesn't like to see companies use the word "bay" in their domain names. Legal challenges will sap your resources faster than you can profit off the name you've chosen.

6. Find a domain name that can be branded by you, which means avoiding generic names and phrases that can easily be copied.

7. Brainstorm names at **thesaurus.com**.

Invest in Domain Names – More Is Better

The title of your product and your domain name are inextricably linked. If the title of your e-book doesn't lend itself to a domain name that's still available, then you need to rethink the title until you come up with one that's a triple threat: It's a catchy title for your product, it lends itself to an easily remembered domain name, and it's part of a brand that you can grow with multiple products at a variety of price ranges, as discussed way back on Day Two.

Once you settle on a domain name, *buy all the similar names.* That includes plurals and different spellings. I purchased dozens of related domain names for *The Millionaire Workout.* Here's a partial list:

- millionaireworkout.com

- themillionaireworkout.com

- millionaireworkouts.com

- millionaire-workout.com

I even purchased **billionaireworkout.com**. I don't think it's possible to buy too many variations. Get as many as your budget and imagination allow.

You can also buy domain names for future products. If you think of a phrase that would make a great title for an e-book down the road, get it now. I own hundreds of domain names. Some I use actively. Some I won't need for another year or so. Some I may never use. I see it this way: If you don't grab it today, someone else might get it tomorrow.

There are two other reasons for getting multiple variations on your domain name. The first is strategic: You can use multiple sites to test different promotions, incentives, and advertising tactics, and then track the sales. The second is commercial: You can lend domain names to other people who're acting as your affiliates. (You'll learn more about affiliate programs on Day Fourteen of the coaching program.)

I take the importance of domain names so seriously that I set up a low-cost registration service for my clients: **ryanleeinternet.com**. Yes, I do make a profit off this service, and in that sense I understand that my advice to register multiple domain names is self-serving. But I also make it easier for you to follow my advice, not to mention making it easier for me to follow my own advice.

One more point about domain names:

Some of you may come up with a great title, but find that someone else owns it. Often, the owner isn't actually using the site, but instead owns it for the sole purpose of selling the domain at a profit. One company, **afternic.com**, sells domain names in auctions. Another, **buydomains.com**, sits on thousands of names that it sells to people like you for a premium price.

Should you buy an existing domain for more than it would cost to create and register your own? It's up to you. If you think you've found the perfect domain name, one that lends itself to a broad range of products within a single brand, it could work out for you. But more often than not, as a businessperson, you should launch your information products with as little up-front cost as possible. That includes getting a domain name for the minimum, $10 or less.

Day Eight • Get Fit

This entire workout will take you about 10 minutes.

Do each exercise for 10 seconds, rest for 20 seconds, then start the next exercise. Continue the cycle of 10 seconds of exercise, followed by 20 seconds of rest, until you've done all eight exercises. This is one "round," and it should take you exactly four minutes.

After you complete the round, rest two minutes (or three minutes, if you feel you need it). Then do a second round.

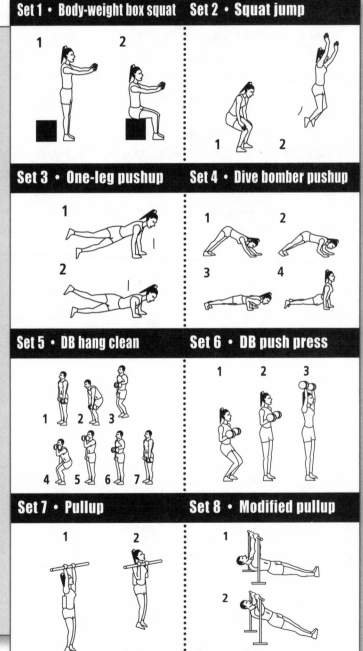

Set 1 • Body-weight box squat
Set 2 • Squat jump
Set 3 • One-leg pushup
Set 4 • Dive bomber pushup
Set 5 • DB hang clean
Set 6 • DB push press
Set 7 • Pullup
Set 8 • Modified pullup

Day Eight • Eat Right
Add a "Cheat" Meal Once a Week

I suppose that someone out there can follow a strict diet without ever cheating. But I can't, and I suspect you can't either. That's why it's perfectly acceptable to relax your diet once a week with something called a "cheat" meal.

The best cheat meal is the one you enjoy the most. Let's say you eat five meals and snacks a day. That's 35 meals a week. If 34 of those meals are part of a healthy lifestyle—lean protein sources mixed with foods high in fiber, vitamins, and minerals—then it's actually good for you to cut loose on the 35th meal, and eat something that no one would recommend as part of a healthy diet.

Personally, I love chocolate chip cookies. There's almost nothing better than a warm cookie right out of the oven. If I thought I had to swear off them forever, I'd be a bitter man. The solution is easy: I have one or two cookies a week as a special treat I give myself. It doesn't sound like much, but believe me, it hits the spot. I tell myself it's a reward, and that's exactly how it feels.

The key is moderation. Two cookies are a treat you can anticipate and savor. A whole box of cookies is a binge. It won't give you any pleasure at all—you'll feel worse afterwards. Same with pizza: Two or three slices once a week tastes like heaven. Eating an entire extra-large pie with five meats and three cheeses feels like desperation.

Maybe you love eating popcorn at the movies. If you know you're going to see a movie on Saturday night, tell yourself that's when you'll have your cheat meal. (It doesn't have to be an entire meal, obviously.) Still, you don't need to gorge yourself to enjoy the popcorn. Order a small size, eat it slowly, and wash it down with water—one of those nice $3 bottles they sell you at the theater. A few glasses of water before your cheat meal can help. (That said, unless you have an impressively expansive bladder, you probably don't want to drink a lot of water before sitting down to watch a two-hour movie.)

Also keep in mind the difference between a cheat *meal* and a cheat *day*. One indulgence a weak helps you stick with your goals. A full day of eating poorly can have the opposite effect. It becomes too easy to fall back into your bad old habits.

Day Eight • Notes and Action Steps

Get Rich

- Jot down a list of at least 10 different domain names you like (including plural versions and different spellings).
- Go to <u>ryanleeinternet.com</u> (you can also do this on sites I don't own), and register *all* of them, or as many as you can afford.

Get Fit and Eat Right

- Perform your workout of the day.
- Schedule one cheat meal into your week.

Day Eight • Notes

_____

_____

_____

_____

_____

_____

9

DAY NINE

M

▼

*Build a web site
with no
computer skills*

▲

W

▼

*Perform your workout
of the day*

*Include more sources
of lean protein in
your daily diet*

▲

Day Nine • Get Rich
Build a Web Site Quickly, Cheaply, and Effortlessly— No Computer Skills Required

Now that you have a string of domain names, you're going to build a site for them. You have two ways to do this:

1. Hire someone

If you can afford it, I recommend hiring a professional. You can get someone to design a nice-looking site with five to 10 pages for about $300. There's no limit to the amount you can spend on Web site development, but I think there is a floor. I once hired a college kid, and although I saved money, it was a nightmare to get him to update the site. It cost me in the long run. That's why I believe you should always go with a designer who's a full-time pro. Check his references and online portfolio. Even someone who's recently launched his business should be able to direct you to sites he either designed or worked on. If he doesn't, steer clear.

Be as specific as you can when working with a designer. The more you streamline the process, the less it will cost, and the better the relationship you'll have with the designer.

Three places to look for a low-cost web designer: elance.com, getafreelancer.com, and guru.com.

2. Do it yourself

You can find hundreds of web-creation software programs, starting with Microsoft Front Page and Adobe Dreamweaver. Each has a learning curve, and it might take you months to get good at any of these programs. You probably want to start with some kind of hands-on instruction—perhaps a continuing-education class at a local college—or at least an online course. Once you learn the basic principles that underlie all web design, it'll be easier to figure out which software program will work best for you.

You can also find Web-based template programs. It shouldn't surprise you to learn that I have one of these at **ryanleeinternet.com**. These sites give you some basic templates to choose from, as well as an editing system to allow you to make changes to your site once you've logged on. Expect to pay anywhere from $5 to $20 per month for a template program.

There's no choice that works for everybody. A template program allows you to put up a site as fast as possible for as little money as possible. Learning to create your own sites takes more time, but gives you a skill that you'll be able to use throughout your career as an entrepreneur. If you get good at web design and find you enjoy it, you could save yourself many thousands of dollars over the years. The easiest choice, if you can afford it, is to hire a designer, with the goal of establishing a long-term working relationship that's mutually beneficial.

Steal This Web Site

No matter which option you choose, you first need a really good idea of what you want the site to look like. No designer can read your mind, and if you expect him to, you'll spend a lot of money on revisions. Even if you're designing your own site, it helps to know what you want, rather than wasting hours staring at a blank page on your computer screen.

Short on inspiration? Make it easy on yourself: Find a site you like, and borrow your favorite design elements.

Start with a simple Google search, using keywords that apply to your ideas for information products. Don't allow yourself to be inspired entirely by the first site you visit. Instead, spend some time clicking through a number of sites. Take notes when you see something you like, paying close attention to these elements:

- Color
- Font (size and type)

- Theme
- Navigation (top, left side, right side, etc.)

- Layout
- How easy is it to get around the site

- Graphics

You probably won't find any single site where you like all these elements. But here's one of my favorite tips: If you find a site that you love, scroll to the bottom of the front page, and see who designed it. You'll often find a link to the designer's site. If it's not there, click through other parts of the site ("About Us," for example) to see if the designer is listed. Corporate Web sites may not list the designer, especially if the company is big enough to have an in-house team in charge of its sites. But if you're looking for ideas at corporate sites, you're probably wasting your time. Whatever you like about those sites could be out of your price range, or involve branding elements that you wouldn't be able to use. Save time and spare yourself frustration by studying sites that sell products like yours.

Easy, Effective Design

A few rules to keep in mind:

- Keep your site basic, clean, and uncluttered.

- Start off with a strong headline that offers a benefit. (Sorry, but "Welcome to my site!" is *not* a good headline.)

- Include an address and working phone number. This builds trust with your customers.

- Make it easy to use your site, using consistent, clearly labeled navigation links.

- Don't make customers work to find your links. They should be in blue text and underlined.

- The text should be easy to read: white background, black letters.

- Keep fonts and sizes consistent. A large blue headline, followed by a small red paragraph, followed by black text with randomly placed blue words induces eyestrain. Your customers will leave before they even know what you have to offer.

- Don't use a Flash intro. Just take them to the text on your home page.

- Keep graphics small. The larger they are, the longer it takes to download your pages.

- Related point: If you decide to include advertising on your site, limit the number of flashing banners or animated graphics. They annoy customers and distract from your sales message.

- Keep the design consistent throughout the entire site. Your graphic elements are part of your brand. If your graphics are jumbled and confusing, your customers will assume your products are messy and poorly conceived.

- Have a method to get each visitor's email address, which you'll use to follow up at a later time. This is the foundation for your online business. (You'll learn the details in tomorrow's coaching session.)

Day Nine • Get Fit

Once again, you'll do the exercises for 15 seconds, rest 15 seconds, and do three rounds of exercises.

But you'll notice a difference in the exercise selection: You'll alternate sprinting in place with a variety of core exercises.

Set 1 • Sprint in place

1   2

Set 2 • Elevated Prone Hip Extension

1   2
3   4

Set 3 • Sprint in place

1   2

Set 4 • Alternating toe touch

1   2
3   4

Set 5 • Sprint in place

1   2

Set 6 • Crunch w/90° knees

1
2

Set 7 • Sprint in place

1   2

Set 8 • Bicycle crunch

1
2

Day Nine • Eat Right
Stay on Track
with a Food Journal

Keeping a journal is not just for teenage girls. It's the best tool you have for tracking your diet and figuring out where you can make improvements. The journal doesn't have to be complicated. Nor do you have to buy a fancy $30 journal with gold letters. My company's nutritionist, Jayson Hunter, R.D., created one you can download for free at ryanlee.com/insider.

A journal gives you the data you need to figure out if you're eating too much or too little. You can see if you're choosing the right foods or the wrong ones. You can see patterns in your journal entries that you might not notice otherwise. You might see that you always slip up and eat the wrong things or the wrong quantities at certain times of the day.

Over the course of weeks or months, if you aren't reaching your goals, the answer can probably be found in your food journal. In fact, studies have shown that many of us have faulty memories when it comes to food. One study showed that overweight subjects forgot half the food they'd eaten in the previous 24 hours. They either forgot something they ate, or underestimated how much of it they'd eaten. The average person underestimates his food consumption by 25 percent.

Other studies have demonstrated that subjects who monitor their diets with food journals lose more weight than those who don't.

Day Nine • Notes and Action Steps

Get Rich

- Choose one method to build a web site (hire a designer, do it yourself, or use a template program).
- Find sites you like, focusing on those with goals similar to yours, and list which elements you like. If you've decided to hire a designer, create a list of design elements you want for your own site, as well as the sites where you found them.

Get Fit and Eat Right

- Perform your workout of the day.
- Start a food log. The easiest option is to the download the free log at **ryanlee.com/insider**

Day Nine • Notes

_____

_____

_____

_____

_____

_____

_____

_____

10

DAY TEN

M

▼

Investigate email
hosting services

Come up with an idea
for a special offer

Place signup boxes on
your site

▲

W

▼

Perform your workout
of the day

Find a good post-
workout drink, and
have it as soon as pos-
sible after today's
workout

▲

Day Ten • Get Rich
How to Turn Email into Money

W hat we've covered in the first nine days is crucial to your success as an online entrepreneur. But if I had to pick one lesson that's more important than any of the others, it's the topic of today's coaching session. Your email list is the lifeblood of your business. It's more important than your product, your Web site, your logo, or the title of your e-book. It's the key to building wealth online.

If you took away everything I have—my money, my Web sites, my products, my business relationships—and left me with just my email list and an Internet connection, I'd still be able to earn a full-time income.

When you have a responsive list, you will *always* be able to earn money. How much money depends on a lot of factors, including some we've already covered: your offers, the perceived value of your products, and the perceived risk to your customers.

You might be surprised to know that the size of your list is less important than the *relationship* you develop with the people on your list.

Let's say you have a newsletter that you send out regularly to the people on your list. A newsletter means one thing to you—it's a way for you to sell new products to your existing customers—but it means something else to the people who receive it. They expect a newsletter to include news. That is, information they can use. If you only try to sell, sell, sell, inundating your best customers with one pitch after another while offering them nothing of value, you will lose your customers. They'll unsubscribe to your newsletter, and your orders will tank.

How to Build a Big, Responsive Email List

Every marketing tip in this book is designed to drive customers to your Web site. Once they're there, your goal is to get as many as possible to join your email list. Here's how:

1. **Make it easy to join.** You want signup links throughout your site, easily visible, on every page.

2. Give a really good reason to join. Just saying "free newsletter" isn't enough. Offer an ethical bribe: Give away free bonuses—a special report, audio download, e-book, or access to private, members-only courses or message boards.

3. Sign up with online newsletter directories, such as new-list.com.

4. Gather email addresses offline. For example, if you're speaking at a seminar or conference, offer handouts or downloads of your slides in exchange for email addresses. If you have a booth at a trade show, give away T-shirts or water bottles in exchange for a business card. (Just make sure it has an email address on it.)

5. Look into co-registration services. These are programs that allow subscribers to join more than one email list at a time. Expect to pay fees ranging from 10 cents to a dollar per subscriber.

6. Team up with other newsletter publishers. You probably know people in your industry who have websites, sell products, and send out newsletters. (If you don't, you soon will; people who do what we do tend to find each other.) Some of these people will be direct competitors to you, but others will sell complementary products. For example, someone who sells exercise equipment isn't directly competing with someone like me, who specializes in information products. You can team up with people like this by offering each other's newsletters. After someone joins your list, you can ask if they'd be interested in also receiving your associate's newsletter. Your associate would do the same. This doesn't work if you're selling competitive products. But if you're offering products that appeal to the same customers without directly competing with each other, this can be an effective way to build your email list as well as strategic alliances with your colleagues.

7. Create a "floating" box with a signup form. These features, which aren't disabled by pop-up blockers, ensure that visitors notice your signup form. Since I started them, they've increased response by up to 200 percent on some of my Web sites. The tradeoff is that visitors to your sites will consider them a nuisance, which is why it's doubly important to offer your customers something of value when they sign up.

Email Newsletter Basics

Many clients ask me if they should create their newsletter in HTML—a format that includes graphics and looks like a Web page—or stick with simple text. I've found that HTML newsletters work best for my list. However, you may find that the opposite is true with yours. You just have to experiment and see which brings you the best response.

I don't know how many software programs you can find for newsletters. There might be hundreds. For most of my lists, I use **www.ezcart.org**. I've also heard great things about **aweber.com**.

Those issues aside, there are some universal features and protocols that apply to all good newsletters.

Unsubscribe: You must offer readers a way to unsubscribe from your list. Most newsletter programs build this into your emails automatically. Don't take it personally when people unsubscribe. Every time you send out a newsletter, some people will unsubscribe, no matter how good your information is.

Frequency: More is often better. I've discovered that my newsletters are only effective if I send them out at least once a week. Even when I send three issues in a week, there's no noticeable increase in people who unsubscribe. But, as I was surprised to discover, there's usually an increase in sales. However, this only works if each issue has solid content.

Best days to mail: I've found that the middle of the week—Tuesday, Wednesday, Thursday—works best for me. But, as with HTML vs. text, you have to test this with your audience.

How you handle content in your newsletter is up to you. Your mix might include tips, interviews, answers to readers' questions, and some straightforward commentary. Just keep in mind that the goal of a newsletter is to get a response from your readers. The worst thing a newsletter can be is boring. Nobody responds to vanilla.

I believe that the personal touch is crucial. Subscribers to my newsletters know about my wife, my children, and my values. It's a great format for telling personal stories about yourself, as long as the stories you're telling relate to your customers and the products you're selling.

And you can't be afraid to speak your mind. As marketing guru Dan Kennedy says, if you're not offending at least one person a day, you're not saying much.

Day Ten • Get Fit

Similar to Day Nine, the focus here is on conditioning. But the mix of exercises includes muscle-builders along with the featured exercise.

Work for 15 seconds and rest 15 seconds per exercise.

Do three rounds of exercises.

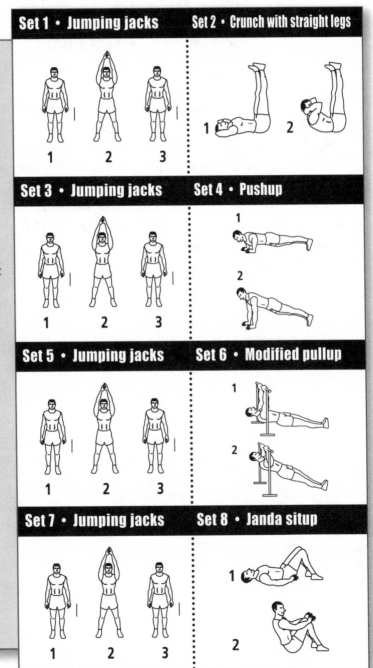

Set 1 • Jumping jacks

Set 2 • Crunch with straight legs

Set 3 • Jumping jacks

Set 4 • Pushup

Set 5 • Jumping jacks

Set 6 • Modified pullup

Set 7 • Jumping jacks

Set 8 • Janda situp

Day Ten • Eat Right
How to Double Your
Workout Results

D id you know what you eat or drink immediately after you workout is almost as important as the workout itself? It has to do with recovery: If your body doesn't recover properly from your workouts, you won't see the benefits. Post-workout drinks are designed to replenish the energy supply your muscles depend on, while also repairing the minor damage you've inflicted on those muscles. The goal is to ensure your body is ready for the next workout. Whether you're trying to lose weight or build muscle, a post-workout drink helps you get there faster.

Ideally, you want to have a post-workout drink within 15 minutes of finishing.

Most of us use "protein shake" interchangeably with "post-workout drink." That leads many people to assume that the key ingredient in the drink is protein. Not so. A good recovery beverage will have two or three grams of carbohydrates for every gram of protein. So if your drink contains 20 grams of protein—which is plenty for just about anyone—you want 40 to 60 grams of carbohydrates.

The best type of protein after your workout is whey, a milk protein that digests quickly and easily. You also want fast-working carbohydrates, such as maltodextrin, which is found in many high-quality post-workout mixes.

My favorite brand of post-workout drink is my own: Prograde Workout (**progradenutrition.com**), which meets the criteria for carbs and protein I just mentioned.

Day Ten • Notes and Action Steps

Get Rich

- Investigate email hosting services, and if you're ready, sign up with the one you like the most.
- Come up with an idea for a special offer you'll give to anyone who signs up.
- Place signup boxes on your site. If your site isn't yet ready, check out sites with goals similar to yours, and see where they place their signup links.

Get Fit and Eat Right

- Perform your workout of the day.
- Find a good post-workout drink, and have it as soon as possible after today's workout.

Day Ten • Notes

_____

_____

_____

_____

_____

_____

_____

_____

_____

11

DAY ELEVEN

M

▼

Set up an account for your online business to receive credit-card orders

The best choice for most is clickbank.com

▲

W

▼

Perform your workout of the day

Eat a good breakfast

▲

Day Eleven • Get Rich
Credit Cards, Security, and
Getting Paid Online

When I first started my online business, about half the payments came via checks in the mail. I had to manually enter all of the credit card numbers onto a printed form and call an 800 number to receive authorization. I was overwhelmed by the paperwork when my business started to take off, spending up to two hours a day just entering orders into the system.

Today, my business is on autopilot. I wake up in the morning and look at the overnight orders, and then go about my day without having to worry about hours' worth of paperwork. And it'll only improve from here: The technology keeps getting better, and the customers are more comfortable using their credit cards on the Internet.

Still, you do have to make some choices before you can sit back and watch the orders roll in.

First, of course, you have to choose to accept credit-card orders in the first place. (Obvious, I know, but I do occasionally get questions from people who're sincere about starting an online business but wonder if there's some way around the credit-card issue. Trust me, there isn't.)

Second, you have to decide if you want to get your own merchant account, or use a third-party solution.

Merchant account: With your own account, you accept payments through a financial institution of your choice, usually a bank. You pay the bank twice for each transaction. First, you pay a flat transaction fee, probably about 25 cents per order. Second, you pay a percentage of the sale price, usually about 2 percent. On a $100 order, the bank would get $2.25, and you'd get $97.75.

Startup costs can range from $150 to $500 dollars, with a monthly minimum of $10 to $50 a month. That is, the fees your sales generate must meet or exceed the monthly minimum set by your bank. If they don't, the bank will take out the balance from your sales revenue.

The benefit of having your own merchant account is that you maintain control of the payments. The downside is higher startup costs and more moving parts. You have to keep a close eye on payments, refunds, and chargebacks.

My merchant account is with a company called Practice Pay Solutions (www.practicepaysolutions.net). I've been using them for over 6 years and I highly recommend them.

<u>Third-party merchant</u>: These companies act as your merchant account. They process your customers' credit-card payments and send you what's left after they take out their percent. That percentage is a lot higher than you'd pay with your own merchant account, up to 8 percent of each sale.

Although you give up more of your sales, there are serious advantages to starting out your business with a third-party vendor. The startup costs are low, and the service is easy to use.

I've had good experiences with these three companies:

- <u>clickbank.com</u>: I recommend ClickBank as your best choice when you're ready to sell your first e-book. You pay a $49 setup fee, $1 per transaction, plus 7.5 percent of each sale. The biggest benefit of ClickBank is the built-in affiliate module, which allows other people (more than 100,000 are signed up) to sell your products. You choose the percentage of each sale that goes to your affiliates, and the company sorts it out from the point of transaction.

- <u>2checkout.com</u>: This vendor has lower fees, but its affiliate option was still in the beta stage as I was finishing this book. You'll pay $49 to start up, 45 cents per transaction, and 5.5 percent of each sale.

- <u>paypal.com</u>: No startup fee, but you pay $20 per month for the service. Fees are on a sliding scale, starting at 30 cents per transaction plus 2.9 percent of each sale. You can sell physical and digital goods.

Each of the three services I recommend allows recurring billing. This is a great feature when you create " --- of the Month" products or membership sites that require a monthly fee.

Tips for Smooth Online Processing

When you get approved for your own merchant account, it's important to maintain a good rating. If you're committing fraudulent or deceptive activities, the bank can shut you down and hold your money.

Also, if you're going to do a big launch that will bring in large sums of money (that is, a lot more than your typical volume), give your financial institution a heads-up. I once forgot to tell my provider, and when I had a big surge in sales, they held up my money for several weeks.

To avoid chargebacks—which occur when your provider gets a complaint from a customer and credits his account, while taking money out of yours—make sure your customers know the name of the company that will appear on their credit-card statement. Tell them on the "thank you" page, which they'll see after a transaction is complete, and in your follow-up emails as well.

Most important of all is something I mentioned early in *The Millionaire Workout* and probably haven't repeated as often as I should: Give your customers more than they expect. Not only should you overdeliver on the product itself, making it better than they thought it would be, but you should throw in unannounced bonuses to make them feel great about doing business with you. Whether it's an extra DVD, CD, e-book, or T-shirt, your goal is to reward your customers with something that has perceived value to them, but wasn't expensive for you to create and produce.

Day Eleven • Get Fit

Use the same protocol you followed the previous several days: 15 seconds of work, followed by 15 seconds of rest.

Do three rounds of exercises.

Set 1 • DB curl and press

Set 2 • DB squat and swing

Set 3 • Feet-elevated pushup

Set 4 • DB squat and swing

Set 5 • Pullup

Set 6 • DB squat and swing

Set 7 • Alternating toe touch

Set 8 • DB squat and swing

Day Eleven • Eat Right
Eat Breakfast

I know this isn't the first time you'd been told that you must eat breakfast every morning. But it bears repeating here, for this simple reason: If you skip breakfast, you'll probably eat more total calories throughout the day. That's what happens when you starve yourself for 12 hours or more. A typical breakfast-avoider isn't hungry in the morning, so she'll go to work without it. She'll try to get by on caffeine until lunchtime, by which time she's ravenous. If she hasn't indulged in a pastry or two before lunch, she'll wolf down the richest, highest-calorie food she can find at noon. She'll probably eat a big dinner, and then continue eating right up to bedtime ... which helps explain why she isn't hungry when she wakes up in the morning.

But there's another consequence to skipping breakfast (or any meal, really): Your metabolism slows down. No food, no TEF. Meanwhile, your body still needs calories to function efficiently. Your brain, heart, lungs, kidneys, and liver don't stop just because you're asleep. Your muscles and skin are still creating new tissues while breaking down or shedding the old. That's why your body functions best when you start refueling it first thing in the morning. If you don't fuel it, your body downshifts. It'll still keep all the important parts operating, but it won't use as many calories in the process. If you're trying to lose fast, or just maintain your current weight, the last thing you want is a slower metabolism.

If that's your pattern, you need to break it. Breakfast doesn't have to be elaborate or fancy. It just needs to be something. You can prepare and eat a solid breakfast in five minutes or less.

One of my favorite breakfasts is hard boiled eggs (whites only; I throw out the yolks), a slice of whole-wheat toast, and water. To save time, I boil a dozen eggs at a time, usually at night, usually while I'm doing other things at the same time, and then store them in the fridge. If I eat four hard-boiled eggs a day, starting the next morning, I'll have three days' worth of breakfasts with just a few minutes of prep time.

Another good choice is peanut butter (get the natural kind, without all the salt and oils added, and store it in your refrigerator). A couple of table-spoons on a whole-wheat English muffin will give you a good start for the day.

If you love cereal, find one with less than 6 grams of sugar per serving. High-fiber bran cereals are a great choice; combined with low-fat or skim milk, you start your day with great sources of fiber and protein.

Try to avoid the biggest breakfast bad-boys—bagels, donuts, pastries. If you have a craving for the sort of things you typically find in a bakery or your local coffee shop, save it for a cheat meal.

Day Eleven • Notes and Action Steps

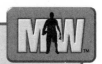

Get Rich

- Set up an account for your online business to receive credit-card orders. The best choice for most entry-level online entrepreneurs is clickbank.com.

Get Fit and Eat Right

- Perform your workout of the day.
- Eat a good breakfast.

Day Eleven • Notes

_____

_____

_____

_____

12

DAY TWELVE

M
▼
Sign up for a
blog service

Create your
first blog
▲

W
▼
Perform your workout
of the day

Include more sources
of lean protein in
your daily diet
▲

Day Twelve • Get Rich
Blogs, Blogs, Blogs

Y ou probably read blogs. You've probably learned from some, while regretting the time you wasted on others. A blog, after all, is only as good as its blogger. And make no mistake, there are a lot of bloggers out there—more than 71 million, according to **Technorati.com**.

A blog (short for Web log, in case you didn't know) can be about whatever its author wants to say. Here's why you need one, if you don't already have one:

- They give you a chance to develop a relationship with your customers, since you'll be providing a steady stream of updated information.

- They give your customers a chance to develop a relationship with you, since most blogs allow readers to comment on the author's posts.

Blogs are easy to use—if you can type, you can blog—and inexpensive to create. You can go to **blogger.com** right now and set one up for free. And you can go to my blog at **ryanlee.com** to see how I use mine. The more you post, and the higher the quality of your posts, the more traffic you'll generate. More traffic means more people become aware of you and your products.

You have hundreds of choices for blogging software. The three most popular and widely used are blogger.com (which I just mentioned), wordpress.com (which I use and highly recommend), and typepad.com.

There's no single formula for a successful blog, but there are some universal principles of good writing that apply to blogging:

- Tell a story. As with your newsletter, the worst sin is to be boring. Think about how to relate your topic to recent stories in the news.

- Write stuff people want to read about. No one really cares what you had for breakfast.

• Ask for feedback after each post. This will not only help improve your search-engine rankings (which I discuss in more detail in another coaching session), but will also give people a sense of belonging to your community.

• Update your blog often. Try for at least twice a week. Any less than that and it begins to look a bit stale.

Easy Ways to Boost Readership

Once you've created your blog, you want to syndicate the information. It can get pretty technical, so I'll just hit you with some of the basics. First, go to **feedburner.com** and sign up for a free account, called an RSS feed. This service (which was recently acquired by Google), allows people to receive emails alerting them to your latest posting.

Next, submit your blog to blog directories on the web, which will provide added exposure. There are hundreds of these, and nobody has enough time to sign up with each one. Start with **www.trafficorganizer.com**, which lists all the blog directories. Make sure you register with the most popular: **technorati.com/blogs**, **blogarama.com**, and **blogs.botw.org**.

Other services allow you to notify other Web sites each time you update your blog. Again, it's a fairly technical issue, but you can make it simple for yourself by signing up with pingomatic.com. It's free, and fairly straightforward to accomplish. Once you're signed up, Pingomatic will send a "ping," or an alert, to other sites when you update your blog.

Here's another way to get more traffic: Go to google.com/alerts. Set up a free account, which gives you an email alert every time someone makes a blog post that contains whatever key words you choose. You visit those blogs, and if it seems appropriate, reply to the post with your keywords. Since the signature line on your reply will contain a link back to your blog, you're sure to get reciprocal traffic.

Day Twelve • Get Fit

Now you'll shift back to a more challenging work-rest ratio: You'll do each exercise for 20 seconds, and rest 10 seconds.

Do two rounds of exercises.

Set 1 • Burpee with pushup

1 2 3 4 5

Set 2 • Jumping jacks

1 2 3

Set 3 • Burpee with pushup

1 2 3 4 5

Set 4 • Jumping jacks

1 2 3

Set 5 • Reverse lunge

1 2

Set 6 • Sprint in place

1 2

Set 7 • Reverse lunge

1 2

Set 8 • Sprint in place

1 2

Day Twelve • Eat Right
When in Doubt, Go with Lean Protein

I've already described many of the benefits of protein, including these:

- It helps you build more muscle mass, especially when you have some immediately after a workout.

- It makes meals more satiating, which helps prevent overeating.

- It requires more energy to digest and break down than other nutrients, which gives you a faster metabolism.

Starting today, I want you to focus on some lean protein at every meal.

Good Sources of Lean Protein

Chicken breast	Turkey breast
Nonfat cottage cheese	Lean ground beef
Kidney beans	Tuna (packed in water)
Skim milk	Egg
Yogurt (low fat)	

Day Twelve • Notes and Action Steps

Get Rich

- Sign up with a blog service (wordpress, blogger, etc.).
- Create your first blog post.
- Submit your blog to at least five blog directories.
- Sign up for google.com/alerts for your most important keywords.

Get Fit and Eat Right

- Perform your workout of the day.
- Choose lean proteins, with at least one protein source in every meal.

Day Twelve • Notes

_____

_____

_____

_____

_____

_____

_____

_____

_____

13

DAY THIRTEEN

M

Write one article, with a resource box that entices readers back to your website

Submit it to five article directories

W

Perform your workout of the day

Tweak your meal strategy to take advantage of the TEF throughout the day

Day Thirteen • Get Rich Got Articles?

So far, I've had you do a lot of writing in these coaching sessions. You wrote a sales letter early on, and you've been working on an e-book. I had you create a newsletter, and right after that told you to start a blog. Now, continuing with that theme, I want you to start writing articles about the topic in your information products.

By "articles," I'm not talking about the type of journalism you see in the *New York Times* or *Newsweek*. The people who write and edit those articles are trained, experienced publishing professionals who belong to huge staffs of men and women with similar credentials.

But you don't have to go to journalism school for the type of article I want you to write.

Your goal is to establish your credibility in your market niche, and to drive traffic to your Web site by gaining wide exposure among people interested in your topic. In other words, you aren't trying to expose your work to an audience of millions, as you would in a mainstream publication. You want an audience of thousands, all of whom are intensely interested in your topic and could be persuaded to buy your products. I spend an hour or two a week writing new articles. I enjoy it, but more important, those articles help my business.

These articles don't have to be 5,000-word essays. They can be as short as 300 to 500 words. Just make sure each one is informative, and try to find someone to edit it before you send it out.

If you're stuck for ideas, try these six quick and easy suggestions, which come to you from Roger C. Parker's excellent book, *Content Catalyst* (<u>designedtosellonline.com</u>).

1. **Biggest mistakes:** What are the biggest mistakes your clients or competitors make? Example: "The 10 Biggest Mistakes Made by New Chiropractors."

2. **Checklists:** "Ten Things to Do before Opening Your Own Shoe Store."

3. **Symptoms:** "Eight Signs Your Marriage is in Trouble."

4. **Resources:** "Ten Business Books Every Plumber Should Own."

5. **Trends:** "Seven Ways the Real Estate Crash Can Actually Help Your Business."

6. **Questions to ask:** "Five Questions to Ask Before Hiring a Babysitter."

How to Make Your Articles Work for You

At the end of each article, you must include a resource box. This tells readers how to get in touch with you for more information. If you give others permission to reprint your articles, make sure to tell them they must include your resource box at the end of the article.

A resource box should include four main components:

- Your name

- One or two sentences that describe your expertise

- Your website's URL

- A call to action

Here's a sample resource box:

Ryan Lee is the world's leading success coach who has helped more than 127,000 people get fit and make more money. To download Ryan's free one-hour seminar, "How to Fatten Your Wallet and Trim Your Waist in 4 Minutes a Day," visit millionaireworkout.com.

Note the specificity of that call to action, and how it entices the reader to click through to my website.

Promoting Your Articles

Let's say you've written your article, had an editor take a look and offer suggestions to improve it, and written a resource box with an irresistible enticement to get readers to visit your site. Now it's time to get the article out where people can see it.

Your Web site: This is the place to start. Place the articles on your site and create links to them from your home page. Now search engines can find your articles, directing people interested in your topic to your site. The more articles you have, the better your odds of being found by the customers you want.

Don't forget to promote each article in your newsletter and on your blog.

Article directories: There are dozens of these online, the sole purpose of which is to list articles. Many of these directories grant permission for other websites and newsletters to reprint the articles stored in their database, as long as they author's resource box is kept intact.

Start with **trafficorganizer.com**, which lists every article database to submit to, and helps you market your article with tips and strategies.

Some popular directories:

- **ezinearticles.com**

- **goarticles.com**

- **articlesbase.com**

- **articlebiz.com**

- **isnare.com**

Complementary sites: Some Web sites will gladly work in synergy with you. They'll print your articles, and give you permission to reprint theirs. Do a Google search of the best keywords for your niche. When you find a site that you think fits this category, send the webmaster a friendly email about your articles, offering free use as long as the resource box remains on each one.

Day Thirteen • Get Fit

Today you'll do each exercise for 20 seconds, followed by 10 seconds of rest.

Do two rounds of exercises.

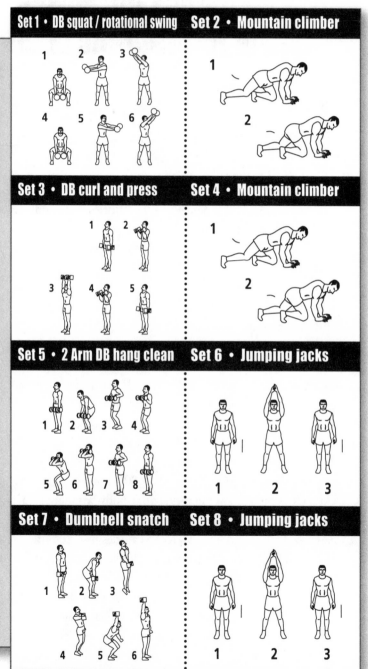

Set 1 • DB squat / rotational swing

Set 2 • Mountain climber

Set 3 • DB curl and press

Set 4 • Mountain climber

Set 5 • 2 Arm DB hang clean

Set 6 • Jumping jacks

Set 7 • Dumbbell snatch

Set 8 • Jumping jacks

Day Thirteen • Eat Right
Unlock the Power
of the Thermic Effect

E very time you eat, your body produces a reaction called the thermic effect of food, or TEF. This is the energy cost of breaking food down into the parts that your body can use. Put another way, TEF represents the calories your body burns to process calories. It's like a physiological service charge, the price your food pays to be part of your metabolism. About 10 percent of the calories your body burns each day are used digesting your meals.

I've already mentioned that protein has a higher TEF than carbohydrates or fat. It isn't even close:

Protein: 25-30% TEF
Carbohydrate: 7% TEF
Fat: 3% TEF

Here's how it works: For every 100 calories of protein you eat, your body burns 25 calories digesting and utilizing that protein. It takes just 7 calories to manage 100 calories of carbohydrate, and just 3 calories to process 100 calories of fat. If you ate a 300-calorie meal that was almost all carbohydrates—a bagel with jam, for example—you'd burn about 20 calories during digestion. But if that 300-calorie meal was equally divided among the three main nutrients, your body would need 30 to 40 calories to process the food. And if it had 200 calories of protein and 100 calories of carbs and fat, you'd burn 50 to 60 calories just from the protein alone.

The TEF lasts several hours following a meal, which means you can have it working for you all day by eating something every two to three hours, with each meal or snack including some lean protein. The pattern of your meals actually does matter: Researchers from Queen's Medical Centre reported that those who ate an irregular meal pattern had a significantly lower TEF than those that eat regular meals throughout the day.

So by increasing your protein intake, as well as the frequency and regularity of your meals and snacks, your body will burn more calories each hour of each day. Your daily workout also boosts your metabolic rate for several hours afterwards, giving you a powerful combination of fat-fighting weapons.

Day Thirteen • Notes and Action Steps

Get Rich

- Write one article, with a resource box that entices readers back to your website.
- If you're confident that this article is ready to be seen by a lot of readers, submit it to five article directories.

Get Fit and Eat Right

- Perform your workout of the day.
- Tweak your meal strategy to take advantage of the TEF throughout the day.

Day Thirteen • Notes

_____

_____

_____

_____

_____

_____

14

DAY FOURTEEN

M
▼
Choose three to four
key phrases to focus on

Submit your site to at
least five major
search engines
▲

W
▼
Perform your workout
of the day

Copy the portion-
estimator chart and
take it with you
everywhere
▲

Day Fourteen • Get Rich
Make Search Engines and
Directories Work for You

I f you want to be successful online, you need to be in the search engines. That is, people have to be able to find you simply, quickly, and easily. There are only two ways to make that happen:

1. <u>Natural search</u>: Someone searches for you and finds you, or searches for your keywords and comes across your site. If you're on the Internet, you can be found this way, and of course it doesn't cost you a dime.

2. <u>Paid listings</u>: You pay to have your site featured for specific search terms. You only pay when someone clicks on your sponsored links.

It gets a lot more complicated than this, of course. Lots of people have come up with lots of ways to game the major search engines, and get more visitors than you otherwise would have. You've probably deleted hundreds of pieces of spam promising to help you do this. Similarly, if you have an active Web site, you've probably gotten countless solicitations from companies that want you to buy paid listings.

Today's coaching session deals with natural searches. Tomorrow's will explore paid listings.

A quick note about terminology: Search engines and directories are often grouped together, but they're different entities.

Directories are categorized and tend to require human editing. Two examples of popular directories:

- search.yahoo.com/dir
- dmoz.org

Search engines are automated. They employ "bots" or "spiders" to crawl through millions of Web sites, compile a list of links that contain your keywords, and then rank them according to their relevance to your search. The three most popular search engines are Google (<u>google.com</u>), Yahoo! Search (<u>yahoo.com</u>), and Live Search (<u>msn.com</u>).

Keys to Getting Listed Without Paying

Search engines frequently change their algorithms to make it almost impossible for people to manipulate the system and get top listings. Companies like Google and Yahoo! hire brilliant mathematicians and computer scientists to ensure their search engines give their users honest results.

There are, however, some basic ways to give your site the best chance to achieve a high ranking.

Submit to every search engine and directory: Every directory and search engine will have a place to submit your site for inclusion. The link might be easy to find ("Add Site," or something similar), but with some search engines you have to dig around. On Google, for example, you first click "About Google," then "Submit Your Content to Google."

Incoming links: The more high-quality links that point to your site, the better your search-engine ranking. For example, a link from the New York Times will hold more weight than a link from a small site with little traffic.

Articles: Write articles that use your targeted keywords, place them on your site, and link to them from your home page. At worst, the articles should be two or three clicks away from your home page.

Create a blog: Search engines love blogs. Keep the content fresh, and you'll gain higher rankings with the search engines. (Tip: Google now owns Blogger; you can bet that blogs using that platform will be noticed by Google's search engine.)

Create videos: Submit them to video sites such as YouTube ... which is also owned by Google. (You'll learn more about video marketing on Day 16 of this program.)

Age your page: If you plan on putting up a Web site in the future, put up a holding page right now. Then let it age. The longer it's been online, the higher your site will be ranked, even if there's no content initially.

Unlocking the Power of Keywords

The more specific your keywords, the better chance you have for success in the search engines. Your site will have a higher overall rank, and the search engines will give your content a higher priority.

Specific phrases—combinations of two or three words, such as "colicky baby"—help you more than general words like "parenting." The single word describes such a broad spectrum of information that you're sure to get lost in the competition, which includes major commercial enterprises. The specific phrase allows people who have a specific problem to find you. And you, of course, sell products that address the very problem these people have.

Two free resources can help you find good keywords

- inventory.overture.com

- goodkeywords.com

My sites have great rankings because I stick with the basics I just described here: links, blogs, fresh content, and specific keywords. Combine that with the rest of the strategies in *The Millionaire Workout*, and you'll see your rankings rise.

Day Fourteen • Get Fit

Do each exercise for 20 seconds, followed by 10 seconds of rest.

Do two rounds of exercises.

Set 1 • Back extension

Set 2 • Seated knee raise

Set 3 • Sprint in place

Set 4 • Jumping jacks

Set 5 • 8-count bodybuilder

Set 6 • Mountain climber

Set 7 • Pullup

Set 8 • Pushup

Day Fourteen • Eat Right
Master Portion Control

R estaurant portion sizes are out of control and growing every year. And as portion sizes get bigger, it's becoming progressively more difficult to figure out what amount of food is enough, and how much is too much. My solution: visualize it.

Proper Portions Made Easy

Write these visual references into your food journal, or jot them down on a small piece of paper you can carry in your purse or wallet. You'll have it memorized soon enough. The first column is the category. The second is the standard serving size. The third is your visual reference. Some types of food make it easy on you. A slice of bread, for example, is a single serving.

CHEESE – 1 ounce (28 grams) = 4 dice

FRUIT - 1 serving = baseball

VEGETABLES - 1/2 cup (120 ml) = 1/2 baseball

PASTA/RICE – 1/2 cup (120 ml) = 1/2 a baseball

FISH/POULTRY/MEAT – 1 serving = deck of cards

PEANUT BUTTER - 2 tablespoons (30 ml) = large marshmallow

MILK/YOGURT - 1 cup (240 ml) = a fist

BUTTER – 1 teaspoon (5 ml) = pat of butter

SALAD DRESSING – 2 tablespoons (30 ml) = ice cube

POTATO – 1/2 potato = 1/2 baseball

A well-balanced meal might include one protein serving, one starch/carbohydrate serving (bread, rice, pasta, and potatoes fall into this category), two servings of vegetables and/or fruit, and a small amount of fat (such as a tablespoon of salad dressing or butter). A bigger person, or someone who exercises regularly and intensely, is going to need more food than someone who's smaller and less active. But for starters, it's good to know what a real portion is supposed to look like.

If that amount of food doesn't look right on your plate, you may want to try eating on smaller dinnerware. It might help, and certainly won't hurt.

Day Fourteen • Notes and Action Steps

Get Rich

- Choose three to four key phrases to focus on.
- Include them as often as possible in your articles and blog posts. If you already have articles written and posted, go back and tweak them to include your most important keywords.
- Submit your site to at least five major search engines and directories.

Get Fit and Eat Right

- Perform your workout of the day.
- Copy the portion-estimator chart and take it with you everywhere.

Day Fourteen • Notes

_____

_____

_____

_____

_____

_____

_____

_____

15

DAY FIFTEEN

M

▼

Set up a free
account at Google

Create a list of five
targeted keywords

▲

W

▼

Perform your workout
of the day

Add the healthiest
foods—almonds, blue-
berries, broccoli, eggs,
salmon, and spinach to
your diet

▲

Day Fifteen • Get Rich
How to Master Pay-Per-Click Search Engines

(Warning: The next sentence is going to read like one of those spam emails you sometimes open because you think they're going to be about something else.)

W ant your Web site to get the top ranking on search engines? You can, and it's 100 percent guaranteed!

The catch? It's not free.

But it is legal and legitimate. It's a type of advertising called pay-per-click (PPC), and all the major search engines have incorporated some version of it.

The benefit of PPC advertising is that you only pay when someone actually clicks on your sponsored link. So if you chose "colicky baby" as your keywords, and someone types that phrase into a search engine, your site will come up as a sponsored result. If no one clicks on your link, you don't have to pay. So, unlike traditional advertising, there's no risk if the ad doesn't work. If it does work and people do click on your link, chances are your sales will more than make up for the cost.

How much you pay depends on the popularity of the keyword you chose—with a range from 10 cents to $15 per click. The higher the demand for that keyword, the more you pay for the privilege of putting your link at the top of a search-engine page. Some companies—including Yahoo!—have a bidding system where you compete with others for your keywords. Others, including Google, take click-through rate and other factors into account many factors to determine the click price you pay.

Get Rich Slowly, or Go Broke Fast

PPC advertising is a terrific way to test your product offers. You can roll out a new program and begin driving traffic via PPC within minutes.

But if you aren't careful, PPC search engines can be disastrous, sucking money from your accounts faster than you can earn it. You have to keep careful track of your results, and how much you're paying to get them.

Let's say you're selling an e-book about weight loss for $19. And let's say you won a bid on a popular search engine for the phrase "diet program." Your price is one dollar per click. But your conversion rate is just 1 percent—that is, 1 percent of the people who click on your link buy your product. So if 100 people who type "diet program" into this search engine click on your link, one of them ends up buying your product. You make $19 from that one sale, but you have to pay $100 to the company that owns the search engine for the 100 clicks that brought you that paying customer. Now imagine the math if you got 1,000 clicks and 10 paying customers. You make $190, but pay $1,000.

That doesn't mean everyone who uses PPC advertising ends up on the wrong side of profitability. Even in the scenario I just described, you could make money if you have a strong product line that generates more than $100 per customer. I know some marketers who have a lifetime customer value of $500. They'd gladly lose $80 on a sale to a new customer if they know their average customer eventually buys $500 worth of products. That's a net gain of $420 per customer over the lifetime of your relationship. The catch is that those marketers need deep pockets to absorb the short-term loss.

You must (must, must, *must!*) know your numbers before you begin spending money on advertising, especially the *lifetime customer value—* how much each new customer is worth to you over the entire time he or she buys your products.

PPC Tips and Tricks

That doesn't mean PPC is the wrong strategy for entry-level entrepreneurs. Here are some simple strategies that could make it pay off for you:

- **Choose niche keywords:** If you go after broad terms like "cell phones" or "computers," you'll pay the highest premium for your clicks. Instead, try more specific and descriptive keywords, for which there'll be less competition.

- **Set a limit:** All PPC programs allow you to set spending limits.

- **Limit total campaigns:** Most PPC programs also allow time limitations. You can run a campaign for a single day, week, or month.

- **Filter your customers:** You don't everyone who's interested in your topic to click on your link. You only want those interested in spending money. If you put the price of your product in the description that accompanies your link, you can discourage window-shoppers and tire-kickers from clicking through. If your copy says, "How to stop your divorce—book costs $29," only people who're willing to consider paying that amount will click on the ad.

- **Bid on a competitor's name:** Let's say Joe Smith has a product similar to yours. If you bid on his name, people who type it into their search engines will see your sponsored link right next to links leading to Joe Smith's. This can be a gray area, legally, as some trademarked companies won't let you bid on their names in search engines.

- **Try "negative" ads:** Some programs allow you to eliminate words from the results. For example, you can filter out users who type the word "free" into a search engine.

- **Be outrageous:** One famous internet marketer (known as the Rich Jerk) might say something like, "You're fat and ugly! Click here to look good like me." It's not a good strategy for the squeamish or faint of heart, but it certainly gets attention and generates clicks.

Pay-Per-Click Resources

There are hundreds of PPC search engines. But you should start with the two major players: **adwords.google.com** takes you to the biggest PPC marketplace on the planet, while **searchmarketing.yahoo.com** is also popular.

Down the road, as you become more comfortable with PPC marketing, you can check out **payperclicksearchengines.com** and **trafficorganizer.com** to find more resources.

Day Fifteen • Get Fit

Do each exercise for 20 seconds, followed by 10 seconds of rest.

Do two rounds of exercises.

Set 1 • Walking lunge, curl, and press

Set 2 • Modified pullup

Set 3 • Dumbbell deadlift curl and press

Set 4 • Modified pullup

Set 5 • Dumbbell snatch

Set 6 • Modified pullup

Set 7 • Burpee w/ pushup

Set 8 • Modified pullup

Day Fifteen • Eat Right
The Six Healthiest Foods You Can Incorporate Into Your Diet Right Now

I'm often asked a simple question by my clients: "What are the best foods to eat?" In the past I'd try to avoid giving a straight answer, since the more you know about nutrition, the more you realize nothing's quite that simple. But eventually I figured out that the benefits associated with some foods really are pretty dramatic, and it can only help to tell my clients which ones offer the most benefit. Right at the top of any list would be the following six, which I've listed in alphabetical order.

Almonds: Great source of protein and heart-healthy fat, along with fiber, riboflavin, magnesium, iron, and calcium. They're also the single best source of vitamin E in the food chain; an ounce of almonds—20 to 25 of them—gives you a day's worth.

Blueberries: The health benefits associated with berries in general and blueberries in particular are staggering. They range from lower risk of cancer to better brain function. A cup of blueberries has more micronutrients than anyone can count, along with 4 grams of fiber and about a third of the recommended daily amount of vitamin C.

Broccoli: If you had to pick one food that exceeds the nutrients found in blueberries, you'd probably pick this one. A cup of broccoli has two day's worth of vitamin C, or close to seven times as much as blueberries. It also give you close to half the vitamin A you need in a day, which helps keeps your eyes healthy, along with 5 grams of both fiber and protein.

Eggs: Egg whites provide one of the best sources of muscle-building protein you'll find. But the real health benefits are found in the yolks. The choline in egg yolks helps your brain work better—the communication system that connects your brain and muscles can't function without it. A single egg yolk gives you a quarter of your recommended daily choline supply.

Salmon: You know that some fats are healthier than others. Omega-3 fats, found in abundance in salmon, are probably the healthiest of all. They've been linked to lower rates of cancer and better heart function. That type of fat is also thought to reduce the level of inflammation inside your body, which is another way to protect your cardiovascular system. Salmon is also a high-quality protein source.

Spinach: Spinach has many of the same benefits as blueberries and broccoli, thanks to high levels of disease-fighting, damage-repairing antioxidants. It also has a powerful effect on the health and strength of your bones, thanks to high levels of vitamin K, calcium, and magnesium.

A Few Words About Fat

You do need fat in your diet, both as an energy source and as an important component of your cells' membranes. It also helps protect your vital organs, gives you healthy hair and skin, keeps your body insulated, and even helps you control your appetite, since you'll feel full longer after meals with some fat.

But not every fat is good for you.

The best fats are those that are monounsaturated (found in olive oil, nuts, eggs, and meat) and polyunsaturated. The two main types of polyunsaturated fats—omega-3 and omega-6—perform a kind of balancing act. Some nutritionists believe that our ancestors grew up with nearly equal amounts of these polyunsaturated fats in their diets. But omega-3 fats have nearly disappeared from the modern food chain. Meanwhile, we find omega-6 fats in all kinds of foods, including vegetable oils. Mayonnaise, made from soybean oil, is a typical example of a recently popular food that provides lots more omega-6 fat than anyone needs. Too much omega-6, unbalanced by omega-3, is thought to lead to higher levels of cancer and cardiovascular disease. While omega-3 fats seem to reduce inflammation, omega-6 fats increase it. With increased inflammation comes a higher risk of heart disease.

Saturated fats aren't as bad as they've been made out to be. There's a wide variety of saturated fats, found in animal as well as vegetable products. Some of them protect us against dangerous microorganisms. Some are good sources of energy. Some are used to build and protect cell membranes. The list of benefits is actually a lot longer than the list of dangers. Even the biggest danger—that the fat will clog your arteries—isn't quite so simple. About a quarter of the fat in arterial plaque is saturated, but half is polyunsaturated.

You don't need to seek out more saturated fat in your diet—you get plenty without trying. You just don't need to purge every gram of it from your meals.

Day Fifteen • Notes and Action Steps

Get Rich

- Set up a free account at Google (adwords.google.com).
- Create a list of five targeted keywords.
- Set a limit of $5 for the day to test your sponsored links.

Get Fit and Eat Right

- Perform your workout of the day.
- Add the healthiest foods—almonds, blueberries, broccoli, eggs, salmon, and spinach to your diet as often as possible.

Day Fifteen • Notes

_____

_____

16

DAY SIXTEEN

M

▼

Set up your affiliate
link on clickbank.com

Find five
potential affiliates
and contact them

▲

W

▼

Perform your workout
of the day

Try to get at least
seven hours of
sleep tonight

▲

Day Sixteen • Get Rich
Unleash the Power of
Affiliate Programs

Imagine hundreds or even thousands of other people promoting and selling your products. Now imagine all of them doing this for free. All it costs you is a percentage of the sales price, which of course you only pay if there is an actual sale.

It's not only possible, it's actually quite easy to do. The concept is called *affiliate marketing*. (It's also known as associate marketing.) First popularized by Amazon.com back in the late 1990s, it's become a staple of online marketing. In fact, for about seven months of my life back in 2000, I helped run a large affiliate directory Web site. This is the job I talked about in the Preface. It was my first and only experience in corporate life, the only time I've been fired, and the only job I really hated.

But as an independent businessman, I've used affiliate marketing extensively, and taught my students how to use it. It's one of the best revenue-generating systems on the Internet.

There are three ways to run an affiliate program. Two are relatively simple third-party systems, which I recommend. Your other choice is to install software and run your own customized program from your own Web site, which is too tricky to discuss here.

All-in-one systems: These programs include shopping carts and affiliate modules. Examples are **clickbank.com** and **ezcart.org**, both of which I mentioned earlier in the coaching program.

Hosted systems: These companies will host your affiliate program on their server. Some will even process affiliate payments for you. The most popular examples are **cj.com** and **myaffiliateprogram.com**.

If you're selling a digital product (like an e-book) and using **clickbank.com** as your merchant (which I recommend), an affiliate module is already built-into the system. That means you're ready to go.

How to Run a Successful Affiliate Program

1. **Offer generous commissions:** You want savvy affiliates pushing your products, and the best partners want to be paid well. Consider giving a commission of *at least* 30 percent of your sales. For most of my products and programs, I offer 50 percent. I go even higher on some programs. This is *not* a time to be cheap. Remember, it costs you nothing. Giving an affiliate 50 percent of a sale you wouldn't have gotten otherwise is a lot better than receiving 100 percent of nothing. Put yourself in their situation: How hard would you work to get 15 percent of a $30 sale, especially if another potential partner is offering 50 percent commission on a similar $30 product?

2. **Make it easy to sign up:** Your site should have links to your affiliate program on every page. A simple link titled "affiliate program" is just fine.

3. **Provide tools:** Create a resource page that includes samples of everything they'll need to sell your product—text links, emails, classified ads, banner ads. Make it easy for them to promote your products.

4. **Offer powerful tracking and management:** Experienced affiliates like to see detailed statistics, such as total hits and conversion rates.

5. **Take care of your affiliates:** Answer their questions in a timely manner, and treat them as valued business partners.

6. **Pay on time:** Set a pay date and stick to it. If you're using an automated system that pays your affiliates (like **clickbank.com**), you don't have to worry about making payments. Other software programs allow you to pay all your affiliates at once using **paypal.com**.

Recruiting the Best Affiliates

The 80/20 Rule—also known as Pareto's Principle—suggests that you'll get 80 percent of your results from 20 percent of your efforts. Applied here, it's safe to assume that 80 percent of your sales will come from 20 percent of your affiliates. If you have 100 affiliates, odds are that 20 will drive most of your business, while the other 80 contribute little or nothing to your bottom line.

A handful of these "super affiliates" might come to you randomly. You have to recruit most of them. Three good ways to do that:

- **Affiliate directories:** Submit your program to some of the dozens of affiliate-program directories. This is the most scattershot approach, but may be your best choice when you're starting out. Two popular directories are **associateprograms.com**, and **affiliateprograms.com**. And **trafficorganizer.com** will give you lists of hundreds more to submit to.

- **Manual recruitment:** You can actively search for potential affiliates by searching keywords related to your topic. For example, if your product topic is singing lessons, you would search keywords like "voice lessons," "vocal coach," "how to sing," and "singing lessons." Visit those Web sites and ask if the owners would be interested in joining your affiliate program.

- **Convert current clients:** Those who already use and enjoy your products could be your best salespeople. I already mentioned the importance of having links to your affiliate program on every page of your Web site. But your customers might see those links and not know they'd be good candidates, and that it's a potentially lucrative opportunity for both of you. So send out an email from time to time telling your customers that they can earn a commission for something they might already be doing—telling people about your products.

You can't underestimate the importance of affiliate marketing, and its potential to build your sales volume exponentially. I recommend focusing 10 percent of the time you devote to your business on this area. Remember, it only takes a handful of productive affiliates can make your entire program successful.

Day Sixteen • Get Fit

Once again, do each exercise for 20 seconds, followed by 10 seconds of rest.

Do two rounds of exercises.

Set 1 • Jumping jacks

1
2
3

Set 2 • Sprint in place

1
2

Set 3 • 8-count bodybuilder

1
2
3
4
5
6
7
8
9

Set 4 • Jumping jacks

1
2
3

Set 5 • Modified explosive pushup

1
2
3

Set 6 • Mountain climber

1
2

Set 7 • Jumping jacks

1
2
3

Set 8 • Sprint in place

1
2

Day Sixteen • Eat Right
Lose Weight
While You Sleep

This might be your easiest session of the entire *Millionaire Workout* system. I can sum it up in three words: Go to sleep! I want you to get at least seven hours of sleep a night. Eight is optimal, but I'll settle for seven, especially if you're currently averaging five or six.

According to Michael Thorpy, M.D., director of the Sleep-Wake Disorders Center at Montefiore Medical Center in New York, "Sleep loss is associated with alterations in hormone levels that regulate the appetite and may be a contributing factor to obesity."

The key hormone altered is cortisol, a stress hormone that has a role in regulating your appetite. When you're deprived of sleep, your body releases more cortisol, which increases your hunger. Research published recently in the *Journal of the American Medical Association* shows that sleep loss does more than increase hunger. It also slows down your metabolism, which makes it more difficult to lose weight, or even to maintain your current body weight.

Tips for Peaceful Slumber

• Stick to a sleep schedule. Try to go to bed the same time each night.

• Avoid stress and stimulation shortly before bedtime, including intense exercise, loud music, or TV shows and movies that get your pulse racing.

• Take a warm, soothing bath (my personal favorite). If you don't like baths, soak your feet in a warm tub.

- Limit the sources of light in your bedroom. These can include LCD readouts from clock radios, video components, and power strips and surge protectors.

- Also cut noise whenever and however possible. Fix dripping faucets or toilets that tend to run. You may not notice the noise a non-digital clock makes when you're awake, but when you're trying to sleep, a ticking clock can be surprisingly distracting.

- If you're susceptible to allergies, minimize the dust in your room by vacuuming often. Wash your sheets and pillowcases regularly.

- Avoid caffeine, soda, and other sugary snacks (and not just before bed—those things aren't good for you at any time of day).

The best benefit of a good night's sleep is the fact you wake up more refreshed, and look forward to starting your day. That can only improve your productivity as you launch your new online business. And losing weight isn't a bad secondary benefit. Who could've guessed you'd get so much out of doing something as easy as sleeping?

Day Sixteen • Notes and Action Steps

Get Rich

- Set up your affiliate link on clickbank.com.
- Submit your affiliate program to five affiliate directories.
- Find five potential affiliates and contact them..

Get Fit and Eat Right

- Perform your workout of the day.
- Try to get at least seven hours of sleep tonight.

Day Sixteen • Notes

_____

_____

_____

_____

_____

_____

_____

_____

_____

_____

_____

17

DAY SEVENTEEN

M

Find three good forums
related to your target
market

Lurk for a few days
to get a feel for each
forum
▲

W

Perform your workout
of the day

Don't let restaurants
derail your
nutrition program
▲

Day Seventeen • Get Rich
Build Your Business on
Discussion Forums

O nline forums can be a monumental waste of time, or a great way to drive traffic to your Web site without any money changing hands. I would've said "drive traffic to your Web site for free," but forums and message boards aren't really free—you're investing your time, and if you aren't careful you might invest too much of it.

Forums are simple enough to understand: They're online meeting rooms for people with particular interests. You register for free, and post messages as often as you like. You can find forums for every interest imaginable, from aardvark grooming to zinc trading and everything in between. It's hard to think of a niche that's too small for an online discussion.

There are two main benefits for visiting and participating in online forums:

- **You'll learn a lot about your target market.** Tune in to what participants are talking about, particularly the questions they ask and the problems they want to solve. It's the perfect place to figure out what your next product will be.

- **It's a great place to build your name.** Nobody starts posting in an established forum and gets accepted uncritically as the voice of authority—unless, of course, you're already acknowledged as the voice of authority on this particular topic. So message boards provide a terrific opportunity to establish your credibility as someone who wants to help members solve problems, and, more to the point, someone whose advice proves to be worthy of attention and respect. But more often than not, this strategy backfires on people who go to forums with the idea of selling products. If you get off on the wrong foot with the forum's leaders and regular posters, you'll be ignored, if not banned from posting again. That's why you need to follow my advice before making your first post.

At this stage of the program, more than two weeks in, you've visited dozens of Web sites related to your topic. Some of them probably have discussion forums. But if you're looking for more, or for whatever reason haven't yet come across message boards specific to your topic, you can find them in seconds with a Google search. Just type in "your topic + forum." For example, if your topic is horse breeding, you'd type in "horse breeding + forum."

Three more places to find targeted, high-quality forums:

- **forums.google.com**

- **big-boards.com**

- **groups.yahoo.com**

Using Online Forums for Fun and Profit

Each forum has its own history, traditions, and levels of acceptable discourse. Most have moderators, one of whom is usually the person who owns the Web site hosting the forum. All have regulars, some of whom will gravitate toward each other and form cliques and in-groups. They might be nerds in the real world, but on this forum, they're the Internet equivalent of the football players and cheerleaders. Nothing will get you banned faster than a dust-up with the moderators and most popular regulars.

I've come up with four simple rules to follow when posting in any forum:

Lurk first: Before you make your first post, read through previous discussions and get a sense of the forum's personalities and protocols. Don't write serious, long-winded posts if the typical forum post is short and sarcastic. Conversely, if people are painfully earnest about the subject, don't jump in with funny retorts that could be construed as dismissive or offensive. The rules really aren't different from those of ordinary conversation, except you can't read the usual cues in vocal tone and body language. So the chances of creating the wrong first impression are very high if you're too pushy, careless, or disrespectful.

Always be helpful: Even if you're the smartest person on the forum and offer a product that will solve most of the posters' problems, you can't just come out and present yourself that way. The worst response you can offer is, "I'm an expert, and if you buy my book, your problem will be solved." Help people by offering honest, practical solutions, without asking for anything in return. Remember, it's a free forum. That doesn't mean the people posting on that forum won't spend money on a product targeted to their interests. But it does mean they're wary of sales pitches. Establish yourself as a reliable source of helpful advice, and forum regulars will eventually get curious about your site and the products you offer.

Create a strong "sig line": Most message boards allow posters to create their own signatures—usually two to four lines of text under your name, which can include a link to your own Web site. Use this space strategically by offering something that's free to anyone who clicks through to your site. Some examples:

- **Free e-book:** This could be something you've already written, or something you obtain at low cost. Ideally, it's a good overview of your approach to solving problems in your topic area, but isn't so comprehensive that people who receive it are less inclined to purchase the products you're trying to sell.

- **Free five-day e-course:** This gives you a great chance to show you can solve problems in a systematic, step-by-step way. All you need to do is create content that you can divide into multiple parts and send separately at specific time intervals.

- **Free interview:** You can interview an expert in your topic area, or have someone interview you. This can be in the form of text or a free audio download.

- **Free special report:** This is usually 10 to 15 pages long, covering a topic that's newsworthy or of particular interest to your target customers. The stronger and more focused the content, the better it functions as a sales tool for your information products.

- **Free teleseminar:** This can be a free registration for a live event, or an audio download of a previous seminar. Make sure the topic is interesting and urgent—"Secrets of the Trade Revealed," for example.

- **Free access to a private membership site:** This can be tricky, since you're posting in one forum with an offer that, in effect, steals members away to another forum. Even if it's a valuable offer, it will backfire if the forum's host sees you as someone who's trying to break up his online community, or siphon off his regular posters.

- **Don't get carried away:** Sometimes you can get pulled into these forums and become a forum addict. If the regular posters sense that you need them at least as much as they need you, they'll be more inclined to see you as a buddy (if not a codependent) and less inclined to see you as an expert offering valuable advice.

And it's surprisingly easy to get sucked into flame wars with other posters, which will destroy whatever credibility you've built. You can't forget that you're the face and voice of your product line. You're the brand. If you're thin-skinned when people disagree with you or criticize your products (and if you have products, someone *will* find fault with them), or too quick to jump into heated, vitriolic arguments that have nothing to do with you, you'll alienate the very people you came to the forum to impress.

You can avoid getting hooked on posting, or too emotionally involved in other people's posts, by limiting your forum time. Set aside some time each week to visit your favorite or most promising message boards, and limit the time you allow yourself to read and answer messages. Set a timer if you need to.

And whatever you do, don't allow yourself to get sucked into silly arguments and personal dramas. Remember, when you're online, you're working.

Day Seventeen • Get Fit

Again, do each exercise for 20 seconds, followed by 10 seconds of rest.

Do two rounds of exercises.

Set 1 • Pushup w/ rotation

Set 2 • Pullup

Set 3 • Body-weight box squat

Set 4 • Reverse lunge

Set 5 • Back extension

Set 6 • Alternating toe touch

Set 7 • Back extension

Set 8 • Bicycle crunch

Day Seventeen • Eat Right
Don't Leave Home Without
This Information –
It Will Cost You Dearly

Eating out at restaurants is becoming the culinary equivalent of a contact sport. If you don't watch out, you can get blindsided by the butter, oils, salt, and sugar restaurants put into food to make it tasty, not to mention the oversized portions.

Some restaurants post nutritional information about the food they serve, and many have started to highlight the healthier choices on their menus. But most of them make it difficult for you to figure out exactly what you're eating. Here are some strategies I've learned along the way to help me make better choices:

- At fast-food restaurants, look for grilled meat or fish, and avoid anything fried.

- In restaurants with table service, choose items that are baked instead of grilled or fried.

- Order sandwiches plain, and add your own condiments, rather than allowing the restaurant to slather on its secret sauce.

- When you eat the sandwich, lose half the bread. Even better, lose all the bread and eat the sandwich contents with a knife and fork.

- Always choose whole-wheat or whole-grain bread, if it's an option. (These days, restaurants that offer it tend to use that as a selling point.) If you're offered a choice of the style of bread—Kaiser roll, bun, panini, baguette—always choose the one that looks smallest. A wrap, for example, probably includes less actual bread than a hoagie or submarine sandwich.

- Choose beans or steamed vegetables instead of fries and coleslaw. Most restaurants will allow this simple substitution for no extra charge.

- If you're in a restaurant in which the waiter brings bread to the table before the meal arrives, politely ask him in advance not to. Having said that, I confess this is a tough choice for me, since I'm a sucker for fresh, hot bread. Thus, you may want to succumb to temptation and enjoy the bread, making it part of your weekly cheat meal.

- If your entrée comes with a vegetable and a potato, ask the waiter to hold the potato and give you a double portion of vegetables instead.

- Choose a salad with dressing on the side. If you're given a choice, pick the simplest dressing offered—olive oil and vinegar, for example, or balsamic vinaigrette. Both provide healthy fats. Avoid creamy dressings.

- Always choose water as your drink.

- If you absolutely must order juice or a soft drink, ask for the smallest size (even if it's the child size).

- Appetizers are often big enough to pass as meals. In fact, you might find a perfectly satisfying meal on the appetizer list, and not even bother with an entrée. If you want an appetizer in addition to your lunch or dinner, make sure you can share it with a companion.

- If you want a desert, split it with someone at your table.

- When ordering eggs, ask for egg whites instead.

- Fish should be grilled without butter or oil. (Sometimes a menu will indicate this by using the word "light" in the description.)

- For pasta, avoid cream-based sauces. Choose tomato-based sauces instead.

Day Seventeen • Notes and Action Steps

Get Rich

- Find three good forums related to your target market.
- Lurk for a few days to get a feel for each forum.
- Once you're comfortable with the flow of the forum, you can join the conversations. Avoid arguments, and be extremely cautious about promoting your products.

Get Fit and Eat Right

- Perform your workout of the day.
- Don't let restaurants derail your nutrition program. The strategies you learned today will keep you from getting blindsided.

Day Seventeen • Notes

_____

_____

_____

_____

_____

_____

_____

_____

_____

18

DAY EIGHTEEN

M

▼

Create a five-minute
video demonstrating
some aspect of your
expertise

Submit it to five
video-sharing sites

▲

W

▼

Perform your workout
of the day

Purchase a box of
high-quality
nutrition bars

▲

Day Eighteen • Get Rich
Video May Have Killed the
Radio Star, but It Can Do Wonders
for Your Online Business

When I first began publishing online, way back in 1998, online video was one of those ideas that sounds great in theory. Unfortunately, it just didn't work. There was no dominant, widely accepted format, and almost everyone had slow dial-up connections. It could take hours to download a simple five-minute clip.

Today, online video works, thank to high-speed modems, more powerful servers and home computers, and the innovations of YouTube and many other sites. It's here, it's here to stay, and it's a medium that can benefit your business.

You can create video clips and put them on hundreds of free video-hosting sites for the world to see. Good video clips can quickly rack up thousands of views. If you have your URL on the video clip, it will drive boatloads of new visitors to your Web site, all of them looking for more.

There's another big benefit of these new video sharing services. They host your video for *free*. Just plug some HTML code onto your site, and you have instant video.

Here are just a few ways to utilize online video marketing:

- **Create screencasts** and publish them as a video tutorial. My favorite screencast program is Camtasia (**techsmith.com**).

- **Edit clips from a live seminar** and submit them to video directories. The seminar highlights will drive traffic to your web site.

- **Perform a webinar,** record it, and spread it virally on the web. A great low-cost webinar program is **gotowebinar.com**.

- **Create a short information video** demonstrating your skill. For example, if you're selling an e-book on home remodeling, you can record a short demo of your installing a sink or putting up new blinds.

- **Interview an expert,** or be interviewed as an expert, and post that. Either interview can be conducted with a digital video camera, available at any electronics store. All you have to do is upload the video online, then post the link on your own site.

How to Create Powerful Video Clips

Most video sharing sites accept multiple formats. YouTube, the leader in online video, has this notice on its site: "YouTube accepts video files from most digital cameras, camcorders, and cell phones in the .WMV, .AVI, .MOV, and .MPG file formats."

That gives you a lot of options, and removes just about any conceivable technical hurdles. That leaves this question: How do you create really good video clips?

- **Outsource when possible:** Unless you're a video junkie, I'd hire someone to film and/or edit your videos. The learning curve for editing software can take a long time, so it's best to pay someone to do it for you. Look in your local Yellow Pages or online classifieds for wedding videographers in your area. They'll often work for a reasonable price during the week, when there aren't any weddings on the schedule.

- **Keep them short:** While there are exceptions, it's usually best to keep your video clips under 10 minutes. Your customers don't want to spend that much time watching an online video, and YouTube and other online services don't accept clips longer than 10 minutes. If you need to have a long video, break it up into multiple clips that run five to seven minutes.

- **Get to the point quickly:** Online readers in general have short attention spans, but with online video, you have even less time to hook your viewers. If you have one really powerful item to share, do it first. Don't wait until the end of the video, because they might not stick around.

- **Beware outdoor audio:** Wind can wreak havoc on audio, as can cicadas, trucks on nearby roads, or just about any other type of noise. So before you make a big commitment to an outdoor shoot, test the sound and make sure you're going to end up with footage you can use online.

- **Don't get too fancy:** In most cases, a $400 video camera is just fine for creating short, promotional clips.

- **Let there be light:** No matter the price of the camera, what matters most are sound and lighting. Your customers have to be able to see and hear the information you're trying to convey.

- **Include your domain name throughout your video clips:** Otherwise, people won't know how to find you.

Beyond YouTube: How to Get the Most Benefit from Your Online Videos

YouTube, of course, is the number-one video-sharing site. As the property of Google, it will continue to grow. But there are other places where you can and should promote your video clips, including but by no means limited to the ones I list below. (Also note that **trafficorganizer.com** features updated listings of hundreds of video-sharing sites.)

- **video.google.com**
- **video.yahoo.com**
- **metacafe.com**

One more big idea: Make sure you register the .TV version of your domain name. So if you already own yourname.com, you should also purchase **yourname.tv**. You can buy your .tv URL wherever you purchased your other domain names, as well as at my site, **ryanleeinternet.com**.

Day Eighteen • Get Fit

Do each exercise for 20 seconds, followed by 10 seconds of rest.

Do two rounds of exercises.

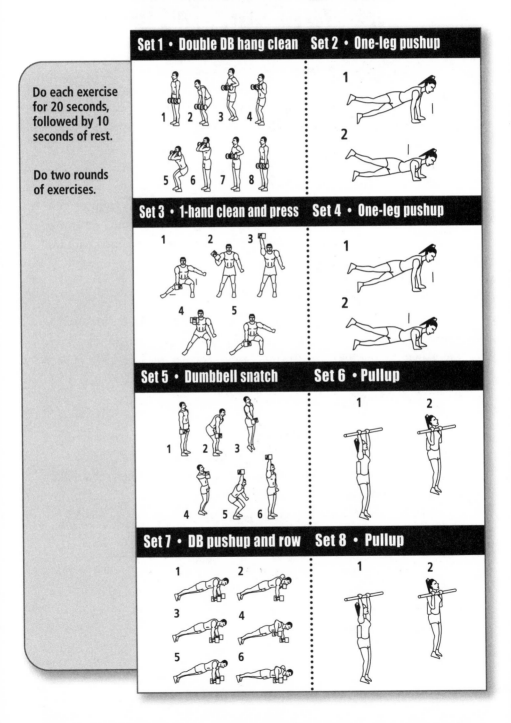

Set 1 • Double DB hang clean   **Set 2 • One-leg pushup**

Set 3 • 1-hand clean and press   **Set 4 • One-leg pushup**

Set 5 • Dumbbell snatch   **Set 6 • Pullup**

Set 7 • DB pushup and row   **Set 8 • Pullup**

Day Eighteen • Eat Right
Beware of Nutrition Bars

I know it's not always easy to bring healthy snacks with you. And I know how few healthy options you'll find on the road—if I wasn't fully aware of how difficult it was before I had kids, I became an expert on nutritional contingencies once they came along.

There's good news and bad news.

More and more convenience stores, airport kiosks, and highway rest-stop food courts now carry protein bars, energy bars, and nuts. And while there are some good ones on the market, many are just candy bars disguised as healthy snacks and meal replacements.

Here's how to tell the difference:

Total calories: Unless the bar will serve as a meal replacement (meaning, you're eating that bar instead of the meal you'd normally have at that time), look for one with 150 to 250 calories. Some of the large protein bars have as much as 350 calories. The lower-calorie bars should hold you over for a couple of hours.

"Red flag" ingredients: The two ingredients you should avoid are partially hydrogenated vegetable oil and high-fructose corn syrup. These two ingredients are useful to food manufacturers, since they're cheap and make food taste better. But they're bad for your body. The first is a trans-fat, which is considered the most damaging type of fat to your overall health. The second is a sweetener that many experts believe could be one of the leading causes of weight gain in America in the past three decades.

Fat: Choose a bar that gets less than 30 percent of its total calories from fat. If you're choosing between two bars with similar overall fat, the one with less saturated fat is probably the better choice.

My choice?

At this point in the coaching program, you can probably guess that I'm going to mention my own product: Prograde Cravers (<u>progradenutrition</u> <u>.com/cravers</u>), in my view, are the best tasting bars on the planet. They're only 180 calories and made with organic ingredients. I usually have one or two a day.

Can't find a nutrition bar? My second choice for a quick and healthy snack is a handful of nuts. I prefer "naked" almonds. Avoid salted and "honey roasted" nuts. "Dry roasted" are only slightly better, since they've been cooked in vegetable oil, a type of fat you probably get too much of already.

Day Eighteen• Notes and Action Steps

Get Rich

- If you have a video camera, create a five-minute video demonstrating some aspect of your expertise, or showing how to do something related to your information product.

- If your video turns out well, submit it to five video-sharing sites.

- Create a link to your video on your Web site.

Get Fit and Eat Right

- Perform your workout of the day.

- Purchase a box of high-quality nutrition bars. If you don't know which ones you like, buy several different bars at a store, have one a day as a snack, and then buy a box of the one you like best that meets all the parameters I described.

Day Eighteen • Notes

19

DAY NINETEEN

M

▼

Create a links page

Find five sites to link to, and contact the webmasters for reciprocal link

▲

W

▼

Perform your workout of the day

Find whole-food-based multivitamins, and start taking one every day

▲

Day One • Get Rich
Choose your target market, topic

A t this stage of the information revolution, I think everyone understands that a Web site doesn't exist in a vacuum. It's not a building on a busy thoroughfare with your company's name in big, bold letters. It depends on other sites to pull in traffic. So all of us know how important it is to have other sites linking to ours. A link on another site is a type of endorsement, a way of saying, "If you like my site, you'll probably like this site too."

But a lot of people, in my experience, still misunderstand how links work.

If your Web site is nothing more than a sales letter—a pitch for your products—it's not going to be easy to get people to link to it from their own sites. Your affiliates will link to it, since they're earning a commission from your products. But it's going to be hard to get reciprocal links.

You have two choices:

First, you can build a links page, which is relatively easy and quick. However, if that's all you do, it pulls people away from your sales letter and sends them elsewhere. Once they leave, it's unlikely they'll come back and buy your product.

The second option is to create a separate Web site with nothing but content. You probably have something like this, since throughout the coaching program I've encouraged you to create a blog and write articles. If you don't, then you need one. This is where people will get to know you. They'll read your blog, see your articles, find links to your video clips, and get a chance to sign up for your newsletter, which means they become part of your mailing list. But the biggest role of this site, of course, is to get people interested in your information products. The links to those sites will be prominently placed on your content site.

Once you have a content site, you've given people a reason to give you reciprocal links on their sites. That is, they're comfortable with the idea of sending visitors from their site to yours. The more reciprocal links you have, the more new leads you can generate for your information products.

Creating a separate site is a lot of work, but also some big benefits:

- **Free traffic:** You'll get visitors from places you couldn't reach with your own marketing. The better your content site, the more links you'll get. The best Web site get thousands of links. If you end up with dozens of incoming links, consider your content site successful.

- **Staying power:** Owners of Web sites rarely take down links once they've gone to the trouble of adding them. I still have links to my sites from people who put them up seven years ago. The longer you keep your content site up and running, the more incoming links you'll have.

- **Search-engine rankings:** Search engines tend to give higher rankings to sites with higher-quality links. You're important to the search engines if other people think you're important enough to link to you.

How to Get More Links

The most common way to start a link campaign is to do a Google search of your targeted, find complementary but non-competitive Web sites, and ask for reciprocal links. Make the appeal to the site's owner personal—if it reads like a form letter, she'll delete it without considering your offer.

If you're asking a stranger for a reciprocal link, you first need to show that you've already done your part. So make sure you show her exactly where the link to her site is. If the site you're targeting has multiple sets of links, ask for the specific spot that would most appropriate.

Next, provide the site owner with the URL you want her to link to—don't leave that to chance. You can also provide HTML code so she can just paste your link into the appropriate place. Make it easy.

A logical question: Why should the owner of an established site give an entry-level person like you a coveted link? After all, nobody wants to clutter his site with hundreds of links. As I said earlier, a reciprocal link is a type of endorsement, and the longer someone operate a site, and the more popular that site becomes, the more careful he is about the links he offers.

One way to get around that is to give someone an award. Everyone likes winning something. You can create your own awards in your niche. It could be something like "Top 10 Horse-Training Sites." Create a graphic that looks like a trophy or medal, and then contact the Web sites to tell them they've won or been nominated for this award. Many will happily place the award on their site, with a reciprocal link back to your site.

Obviously, you can't do this if the sites you're targeting are too big to care what you think of them. A mega-site like espn.com isn't going to play ball with someone who made up an award to get a reciprocal link.

Which brings me back to the importance of patience. Unless you're already well-known in your field, it's going to take time to build credibility, move up in search-engine rankings, and draw high-quality links to your site.

That doesn't mean you should sit back and hope the audience finds you. That's no way to run a business. You can, however, outsource the search for appropriate links you can get now. Search for a qualified freelancer at <u>elance.com</u>, <u>guru.com</u>, and <u>brickworkindia.com</u>.

Beware of Link-Farm Scams

Lots of unscrupulous companies troll the Internet looking for easy prey. And if you have new sites, you're seen as fresh meat. One common scam is offering you thousands of links overnight. These scams are commonly known as link farms.

Wikipedia defines a link farm as "any group of Web pages that all hyperlink to every other page in the group. Although some link farms can be created by hand, most are created through automated programs and services. A link farm is a form of spamming the index of a search engine."

If you sign up with a link farm, you'll probably get blacklisted from search engines. So stay away. If it sounds too simple and easy, it is.

Day Nineteen • Get Fit

Do each exercise for 20 seconds, then rest for 10 seconds.

Do three rounds of exercises.

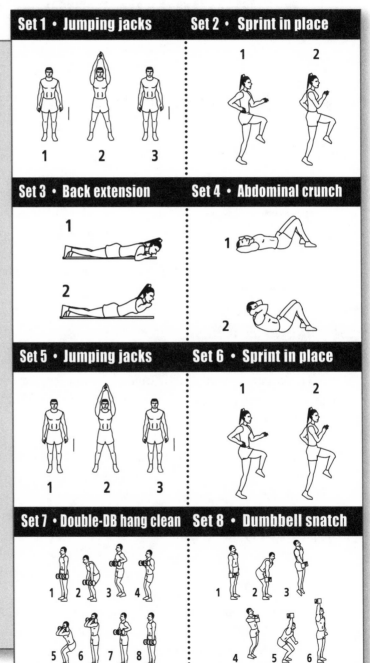

Day Nineteen • Eat Right
Getting Your Fruits and Veggies

I have to admit it: I've never been a huge supplement guy. I've always believed you can get most of your vitamins and nutrients from eating real food. My attitude hasn't changed, but the food has. It's more processed, and there's more risk posed by the pesticides. The nutrients you think you're getting might not be there.

So, while I *used* to promote eating 10 servings a day of fruits and vegetables, I now warn my clients that even that might not be enough. You can be part of the tiny fraction of Americans who eat all 10 recommended servings of fruits and vegetables a day, and yet you *still* may be deficient in certain nutrients.

That's why I now tell my clients to supplement with a whole-food-based multivitamin.

Synthetic vs. Natural

Synthetic vitamins are created through chemical processes, whereas natural vitamins are derived directly from plants or other materials. Most vitamins you find on the store shelves are synthetic, which is one reason they're so inexpensive.

The biggest downside to synthetic vitamins is that, in many cases, you don't get the nutrients you think you're getting. A really cheap pill may not break down properly. Since you can only use what gets absorbed before the pill passes out of your system, all your savings on the inexpensive vitamins get flushed away—literally. But even if the pill breaks down properly and completely, the synthetic nutrients may not be absorbed and utilized.

A whole-food vitamin, on the other hand, has nutrients that come directly from fruits and vegetables. That makes them more readily absorbed and utilized by the body.

That's why, when I started my own nutrition-products company, Prograde, I wanted our vitamins to come from whole foods. I also made sure that the fruits and vegetables we used were grown in ideal conditions, using as few pesticides as possible. I confess my motives were slightly selfish: I wanted to know the vitamins my wife and I take were made from the best components, grown in the best conditions.

The vitamins we take are called VGF 25+ for Men and VGF 25+ for Women. You can find them at **progradenutrition.com**.

Most of the benefits from a healthy diet will come to you from whole foods. But a good multivitamin, made from whole foods, makes sure you don't miss out on any important nutrients.

Day Nineteen • Notes and Action Steps

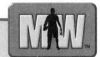

Get Rich

- Create a links page.
- Find five sites to link to, and contact the webmasters for reciprocal link.

Get Fit and Eat Right

- Perform your workout of the day.
- Find whole-food-based multivitamins, and start taking one every day.

Day Nineteen • Notes

_____

_____

_____

_____

_____

_____

20

DAY TWENTY

M

▼

Write down an idea for a viral-marketing project that will get attention

Get your video, e-book, or special report into circulation

▲

W

▼

Perform your workout of the day

Purchase an EFA supplement, and take the recommended portion every day

▲

Day Twenty • Get Rich
Go Viral

V iral marketing has an unfortunate name. The goal is to get other people—people who aren't working for you and don't personally profit from your work—to pass along your marketing message. The "pass along" part is how it came to be called "viral," although it's hard to argue that people pass diseases to each other with the same enthusiasm.

The first well-known example of viral marketing was Hotmail, the email service that launched in July 1996. When people signed up for free Hotmail accounts, the bottom of every email they sent would include a link back to hotmail.com, inviting the recipients to open free accounts of their own. Word spread quickly, and in just 17 months Hotmail had some 8.5 million subscribers. That got the attention of Microsoft, which snapped it up for $400 million.

And that was in the dark ages of the Internet boom. A decade later, innovative marketers are using countless modalities and media to launch their own viral marketing campaigns.

My Smooth(ie) Experience

One of my earliest successes in viral marketing was an e-book called *Smoothies for Athletes*. It had 130 smoothie recipes (all of which tasted great, in my humble opinion), with complete nutritional information for each one.

I encouraged people to give copies of the e-book to family and friends.

I also allowed resell rights. This gave anyone the ability to sell my e-book and keep all the profits. I knew other Internet marketers were looking for new products to sell to their customers, and a lot of them jumped at the chance for something they could sell at no cost to them. The savviest marketers packaged *Smoothies for Athletes* with their own products and services, using my e-book as a free bonus.

You're probably wondering why I would give it away. It was, after all, a product that had real commercial value. On top of that, I'd worked hard on it, and was proud of what I created. This wasn't the marketing equivalent of a garage sale.

Here's why I did it: Throughout the e-book I'd included links back to my Web sites. The more people who saw the e-book and clicked on the links, the more chances I had to generate business for my other products.

Boy, did it work. And it keeps working. Today, four years later, there are tens of thousands of copies of Smoothies for Athletes floating around the Web, and they're still driving new traffic back to my sites.

New Viral Campaigns

If I were going to try the same thing today, I'd use online video. In fact, I have used it, although not for my own business. I was touched by a three-minute video called "Free Hugs," which I saw on YouTube. I sent it out to my mailing list. (Do your own search and watch it. You'll see why I was moved.) The last time I checked, the video had already been viewed more than 15 million times.

Of course, that's just one video, and there are millions of videos on YouTube alone. Only a handful become truly viral and get seen by millions of people. But you don't need millions to see yours. You might profit tremendously from a few hundred, or even a few dozen, if the people who see it are your target customers and send it along to other customers who need your products and services.

I covered videos in more details on Day Sixteen, so I won't repeat all that information here, except to remind you of the top video-sharing sites:

- youtube.com
- video.yahoo.com
- video.google.com
- metacafe.com

And don't forget about trafficorganizer.com, which can help you organize your entire viral campaign.

Down 'n Dirty Viral Tips

Make it interesting: Boring reports and videos don't become viral. People only share it if it's exciting, thought-provoking, and/or uniquely informative.

Keep it short: Nobody's going to share a report or an e-book that's longer than 50 or 60 pages, or a video that runs past the five-minute mark.

Keep your advertising subtle: You can include a short, promotional intro, along with a link back to your site. Or you use a watermark that includes your URL. (Someone sharing the clip might be able to edit out your intro or delete your link, but a watermark goes onto every frame of the video and can't be removed.) But if your video is a pure advertisement, with no informational or entertainment value, it won't become viral unless it's so bad people send it around just to make fun of it. And that's far worse than getting no attention at all.

Help spread the virus: Put your video on your Web site, and give people tools to share it with others on sites such as **digg.com, furl.net, del.icio.us,** and others.

Day Twenty • Get Fit

Do each exercise for 20 seconds, then rest for 10 seconds.

Do three rounds of exercises.

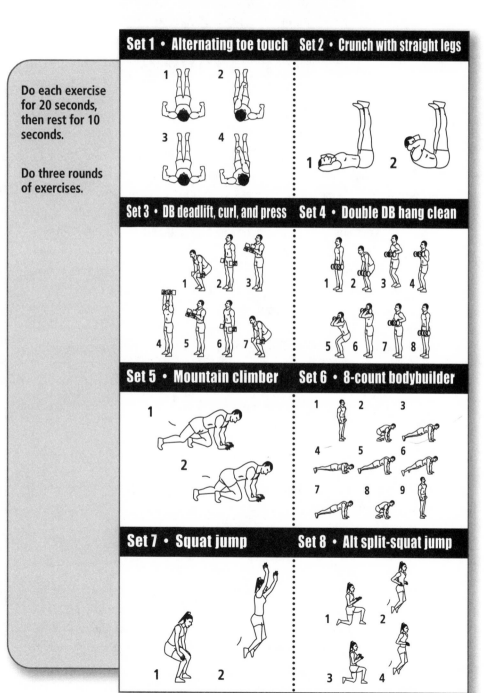

Set 1 • Alternating toe touch Set 2 • Crunch with straight legs

Set 3 • DB deadlift, curl, and press Set 4 • Double DB hang clean

Set 5 • Mountain climber Set 6 • 8-count bodybuilder

Set 7 • Squat jump Set 8 • Alt split-squat jump

Day Twenty • Eat Right
Essential Fats:
They Aren't Optional

Yesterday I told you about multivitamins, a nutritional supplement I take and recommend you take as well. Today, I want to mention a second supplement that's so important it's essential. In fact, the importance is right there in the name: essential fatty acids.

If a nutrient is "essential," it means your body can't make it from other nutrients, and you must have it in your diet. Two polyunsaturated fats are considered essential: omega-3 and omega-6. As I said in the Day Fifteen coaching session, most of us get plenty of omega-6 fats, but it's hard to get an equivalent amount of omega-3 unless we eat a lot of fish (I mentioned salmon) or we get our beef from grass-fed cattle. (Wild grasses have lots of omega-3 fat, which is why meat from grazing animals has more of it than meat from grain-fed livestock.)

Two omega-3 fats—DHA and EPA—have a long list of health benefits attributed to them, including these:

- Improved concentration and memory
- Protection for cell membranes
- Healthy nervous-system function
- Improvement in cholesterol levels
- Support for a strong immune system
- Relief of PMS symptoms
- A healthy heart
- Stronger joints

Since it's hard to get enough omega-3 fat in your meals, and since no health-conscious person wants to pass up the benefits associated with DHA and EPA, many of us take supplements. Fish-oil capsules are the most popular. And, as you probably guessed, my company makes just a supplement: EFA Icon (**progradenutrition.com/icon**).

Day Twenty • Notes and Action Steps

Get Rich

- Write down an idea for a viral-marketing project that will get attention and lend itself to pass-along readership or viewership.
- Make a list of steps you'll take to get the video, e-book, or special report into circulation.

Get Fit and Eat Right

- Perform your workout of the day.
- Purchase an EFA supplement, and take the recommended portion every day.

Day One • Notes

_____

_____

_____

_____

_____

_____

_____

_____

_____

_____

21

DAY TWENTY ONE

M

▼

*Sign up for five
social-networking sites,
and create a profile
for yourself
on each one*

▲

W

▼

*Perform your workout
of the day*

*Keep this book on your
nightstand, and
re-read it whenever
you need motivation*

▲

Day Twenty One • Get Rich
The Day After Tomorrow:
Marketing for the Future

I n the beginning, what we now call the Internet was a network known only to scientists and military planners, a way for them to share the kind of information you and I didn't need to know. By the time everyone had heard of the Internet, it was a top-down and bottom-up medium: The biggest and smallest content providers were doing exactly that—providing content to anyone who wanted it. Readers had a lot more interaction with the providers than ever before, but it was still one-way communication, from the person creating content to the people using it.

Now there's a new dynamic online, often referred to as Web 2.0. Content is produced and shared by communities of volunteers. Wikipedia, for example, allows anyone who registers to create or edit entries. The rest of the community modifies the entries, including edits of the edits, until the content reaches the community's standards for accuracy, clarity, neutrality, and so on. People who try to use the online encyclopedia for personal pro-motion quickly realize that it's hard to get away with it—the community is quick to find and either edit or eliminate that kind of information.

Social-networking sites are another phenomenon that stress community above all else. You can—and should—use social networks to promote yourself and market your products. While each site has its own features and customs, there are some basic steps you can take to join in:

- **Create a free account:** Most sites allow you to register for free, so set up an account. Take advantage of the free exposure and search-engine placement these accounts can get you.

- **Don't be bashful:** If the site allows you to create a full profile, do it. Add photos if you can, as well as descriptions of your products, if that's allowed.

- **Post your links:** Social-networking sites like myspace.com allow you to add links back to your own sites. You can also use bookmarking sites (like digg.com) to link back to articles and blog posts on your own sites.

- **Post comments:** I discussed this earlier in the coaching program, but it applies here as well. Leave comments wherever you can, with your signature line offering a link back to your main Web site. Just make sure your comments are relevant, and won't be construed as spam.

Social-Networking Sites

- <u>myspace.com</u>: the most popular, with more than 180 million registered users

- <u>friendster.com</u>: another well-known social site, with close to 30 million users

- <u>43things.com</u>: you can share your goals and dreams with other 43things members

Tagging and Bookmarking

- <u>www.digg.com</u>: a combination of social networking, tagging, blogging, and syndication

- <u>furl.net</u>: social-bookmarking site that allows you to recommend other Web sites

- <u>del.icio.us</u>: another popular social-bookmarking site

- <u>squidoo.com</u>: create a "lens"—a page that allows you to share information about any topic. It's new but quickly gaining in popularity.

- <u>technorati.com</u>: a search engine for blogs

Miscellaneous

- <u>craigslist.com</u>: extremely popular free classified-ad Web site

- <u>frappr.com</u>: create a social map for all of your members

- <u>flickr.com</u>: share photos with millions of other people

What the Future Holds ...

It's really an exciting time to market your self online. As soon as you feel you've gotten ahead of the curve, you realize you've fallen behind an entirely different curve. There's always something new to learn about marketing your business.

One of my favorite sites for keeping up with the changes is **go2web20.net**, a directory of all these cutting-edge sites.

Also, make sure to use **trafficorganizer.com** to manage your ongoing marketing campaigns.

That brings us to the end of the 21-day coaching program. You've learned a lot, and you've done a lot, but you know that most of the real work is still ahead of you. That's why the bonus section that follows Day Twenty-One gives you a blueprint for a lifetime of profits, fitness, and healthy nutrition.

Day Twenty One • Get Fit

This entire workout will take you about 10 minutes.

Do each exercise for 10 seconds, rest for 20 seconds, then start the next exercise. Continue the cycle of 10 seconds of exercise, followed by 20 seconds of rest, until you've done all eight exercises. This is one "round," and it should take you exactly four minutes.

After you complete the round, rest two minutes (or three minutes, if you feel you need it). Then do a second round.

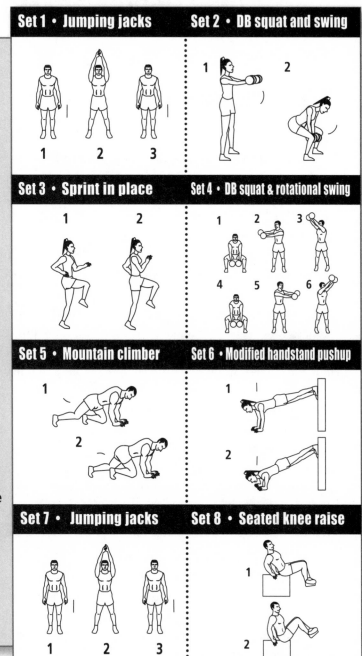

Set 1 • Jumping jacks

1   2   3

Set 2 • DB squat and swing

1   2

Set 3 • Sprint in place

1   2

Set 4 • DB squat & rotational swing

1   2   3
4   5   6

Set 5 • Mountain climber

1
2

Set 6 • Modified handstand pushup

1
2

Set 7 • Jumping jacks

1   2   3

Set 8 • Seated knee raise

1
2

Day Twenty One • Eat Right
Eating Healthy for Life

By today, you probably look better. You've probably lost a few pounds, or at least tightened up your waistline. (Not everyone has weight to lose, of course.) I'm going to guess you feel as if you have more energy throughout the day, you sleep better at night, and you feel a lot better about yourself in general.

You worked hard, and you deserve to feel proud about what you've accomplished. But now you face an even tougher challenge: how to keep it going for the rest of your life. You'll have setbacks, of course. Maybe you eat or drink too much at Cousin Suzie's wedding, or you let yourself go on that two-week vacation in Hawaii that you've been fantasizing about for years.

I'm not talking about those. They're easy to deal with—just get back on the horse. Go back to your exercise and nutrition program, and don't worry about a day or even a month of regressive habits. The health you enjoy for the rest of your life isn't compromised by slip-ups. Your habitual behaviors—what you do most of the time—is what matters.

And if you ever slip up so severely that you feel you have to start over? That's okay. Just remember what you learned in *The Millionaire Workout*: Success comes to you in small, digestible pieces. There's always a step-by-step process that gets from where you are now to where you want to be. It really is the small steps that add up over time to the biggest improvements.

The Millionaire Workout Is Your Lifetime Coach

Remember, *The Millionaire Workout* is your book. You can read it as many times as you want. I have hundreds of books in my personal library, and find myself thumbing through them over and over to refresh my brain on the topic. You can use your re-readings as subtle reminders ... or swift kicks in the butt. Heck, if you remember me as your butt-kicking coach, I'll take it as the highest compliment.

Day Twenty One
Notes and Action Steps

Get Rich

- Sign up for five social-networking sites, and create a profile for yourself on each one.

Get Fit and Eat Right

- Perform your workout of the day.
- Keep this book on your nightstand, and re-read it whenever you need motivation, inspiration, or that swift kick I just mentioned.

Day One • Notes

_____

_____

_____

_____

_____

_____

_____

_____

_____

_____

Bonus Coaching Session

DAY TWENTY TWO AND BEYOND...

L et me be the first to offer you congratulations for completing the 21-day coaching program. Believe it or not, you're way ahead of just about anybody else who wants to do the things you've already begun doing. Very few people take any action to change their course in life and reach their goals. Even fewer go as far as buying a book that promises to tell them how to do it. And only a fraction of those will follow through and complete all the steps in the program.

In fact, if I had to guess right now, I'd say that only a minority of those who buy *The Millionaire Workout* will finish it. You're now part of a very small group—a group that includes me and most of the truly successful entrepreneurs in the world today.

The first 21 days are just that—the first steps, the beginning of your career in information marketing. Now I'm going to tell you what to do on Day Twenty-Two, and beyond.

How to Get Rich, and Stay Rich

Not everyone who creates and markets information products online will get rich. It's mathematically impossible for it to work out that way. Some will, of course. I hope you're one of them, if that's your goal. Some will be happy to create a nice side income, and that's great. Some will be disappointed. I'd like to say that everyone who follows my program will belong to the first category, but it can't possibly work out that way. Your ultimate success depends on your talent, the size and spending habits of the market you've decided to target, and the amount of competition within that market.

The entire point of the coaching program was to get you to create and market a single product. If you stop there, you'll get whatever that single product brings you. Chances are it won't bring you wealth.

Real success comes when you develop a passion for creating and marketing information products, do it full-time and with all your creative energy, and build your business year after year. If that happens, the amount of money you can make is unlimited.

Just look at me: A few years ago, I was a gym teacher in the Bronx. Now I have complete financial independence. I didn't take any special classes that taught me how to do this, I don't have any unique computer skills, and you already know that my master's degree is in exercise science, not business administration.

I worked hard, of course, but that was easy, since I love what I do. If I had to pick one thing that sets me apart, it's the fact that I created valuable products and programs for my customers and clients.

Since no single product or program can solve every problem or meet every need, the key to your success is to create products in different forms, with different price points, to solve the problems of customers with different needs and different resources they're willing to spend to address those needs.

That's why your most promising strategy is to create your own information empire. It will probably include many of these types of products:

- **Books on CD (or audio download):** You can read your own book and record it to a CD, or offer it as a downloadable MP3.

- **Interview on CD (or audio download):** Record interviews with other experts in your market niche, and offer them as a CD, or a multiple-CD set.

- **Interviews (text):** Have the interviews transcribed into a book, e-book, or manual.

- **Case studies on CD (or audio download):** Interview other people who have achieved success in your target market.

- **Case studies (text):** Have the case studies transcribed and put them into a book, e-book, or manual.

- **Workshop or seminar on DVD:** Do a live lecture or demonstration, and record the full program on DVD.

- **Workshop or seminar on audio CD:** Do a live lecture or demonstration, and record the full program on audio CD.

- **Workshop or seminar (big kit):** Combine the audio CDs and DVDs of your live event, and now you have an expensive kit to sell. As a bonus, you can also have all the audio transcribed and include that text as a follow-along manual.

- **Book from the public domain:** Find publications that have expired copyrights. You can reprint them and keep 100 percent of the profits.

- **Private-label products:** You can purchase the rights to resell information products, and put them under your own label or brand.

- **Resell or reprint rights:** Purchase resell or reprint rights of products to sell to your customers—easy profit with very little work on your part.

- **Build a membership site:** This is my favorite information product. Charge yearly or monthly fees to allow access to your best content online. (For an example, check out one of mine: **membersitebootcamp.com**.)

- **Coaching program:** Offer monthly coaching programs, which give clients private phone conversations with you, group teleseminars, or some combination.

- **"Best of" product:** Combine all of your best articles and/or interviews into a Best of ... book or kit.

- **Teleseminars on CD (or audio download):** Promote a live teleseminar, and sell the recordings on audio CD or as an audio download.

- **Screenshot videos:** Use a program such as camtasia (techsmith.com) to record your computer screen. This is great for software tutorials.

- **Live bootcamps:** Run a multiday event in your market niche. Bring in guest speakers, and take a percentage of all the back-of-the-room product sales. I know some marketers who make seven figures with a single weekend-long bootcamp.

- **Resource directory:** Compile a list of resources in your target market—vendors, wholesalers, Web sites, etc. You can sell it as a CD, downloadable file, or printed book.

- **Software:** Hire a programmer to build a software program to your specifications, with unique benefits to your customers and clients. Or you can do like Bill Gates, and buy an existing software program. In his case, it was an operating system called 86-DOS, which he then licensed to IBM, making it the default operating system for personal computers before most people had even heard of PCs. Talk about getting in on the ground floor!

These ideas are just a sample of what you can do with information products. That's what I love about this business—you can always come up with new products, or new ways to package existing products. You might even create an entire new category of products, and I'll have to hire you as my personal coach.

How to Stay Fit Forever

Now that you've learned *The Millionaire Workout exercise* system, you need to keep doing what you've learned. Just about all the benefits of exercise come from what you do habitually, not what you did for a while before you stopped.

The system was created with the idea of giving you the biggest benefits in the least amount of time. If you can't spare 15 minutes, you know you can get a great workout in a fraction of that time. Remember, all it takes is four minutes to do a round of exercises

If you like your workouts set up for you the way they are in the coaching program, check out my home coaching program, which includes a newsletter featuring brand-new workouts sent to your mailbox every month. Just go to **ryanlee.com/insider** for more information.

Keep Up the Great Work

Taking you though this coaching program has been my sincere pleasure. I hope the benefits will greatly improve the quality of your life, now and in the future. If you enjoyed the experience, please pass the word about this book.

Warmest Regards,

Ryan Lee
The Millionaire Workout

—Index—

—Notes—

—Notes—

—Notes—

—Notes—

—Notes—

—Notes—

—Notes—

_____

_____

_____

_____

_____

_____

_____

_____

_____

_____

_____

_____

_____

_____

_____

_____

_____

_____

_____

_____

—Notes—

Now, You can Receive the *Millionaire Workout Insider* Coaching Program: a Up-to-the-Minute Information-Packed Newsletter and Audio Coaching CD Delivered to your Door Every Month...

FOR FREE!*

Because the Internet changes every day and I am always learning new health & fitness strategies to stay in peak condition, it's simply not feasible to write a new edition of the book every few weeks. So I did something even better that will help you – big time!

Every 4 weeks, I take the latest most powerful breakthroughs – and pour them into an easy to read, straightforward printed newsletter. Plus, I interrogate other guest coaches and go into excruciating detail about these breakthroughs - and put that information on an audio CD.

You will receive these __latest__ cutting-edge techniques to help make you more passive income while keeping you in the best physical shape of your life.

No fancy packaging or graphics. *The Millionaire Workout Insider* is straight to the point and, just like this book, 100% fluff-free.

It's just like hiring me as your personal success coach to make sure you are continuing on the path of greatness.

And I am doing something unheard of for a coaching program. See all the details on how the program really doesn't cost you a penny.

You are going to be blown away!